DISTURBED

DISTURBED

JESSICA CLEGHORN

LIBRARY OF CONGRESS CONTROL NUMBER: 2012924273

ISBN: HARDCOVER   978-1-4797-6029-9

SOFTCOVER   978-1-4797-6028-2

EBOOK   978-1-4797-6030-5

This book was printed in the United States of America.

To order additional copies of this book, contact:

Xlibris Corporation

1-888-795-4274

www.Xlibris.com

Orders@Xlibris.com

126787

Fordy, thank you for reminding me that sarcasm is a way of life. Love you, you crude SOB!

Samantha: you are my soul mate. The cover is PERFECT. Stay bitter, my love!

Shauna: With love I say, GET. A. NEW. PHONE.

Bryan and Cathy: I couldn't ask for better loving parents. I love you so much.

And Grey . . . you're still my Pooka. Never forget the frolicking hippos.

CONTENTS

Classification of My Disorders, Symptoms, and Consequences of
    My Eating Disorder 11
Early Years and Development of My Eating Disorder 16
The Unwanted Rite of Passage, Abuse of Narcotics, and
    My First Lover, the Mirror.. 21
My Binging, Purging, and Fasting Habits... 24
Body Image.. 28
Wanting to Look Unhealthy: Bitter for Being Unhealthy 30
Self-Mutilation.. 33
Insomnia.. 35
Normality 39
A Few Things to Clear Up: Being a Pariah 42
Alone.. 45
Grey.. 47
Recovery, Recovered, Triggers... 54
CCU and Suicide Attempt.. 58
Returning Home, the Escalation of My Eating Disorder, Therapy,
    "Reminder of a Necklace Incident" 63
St. Mary's College of Maryland... 71
New Friends and Support... 80
Back to Therapy 84
Residential Treatment 89
Epilogue 103

Dear Mom and Dad,

I'm sorry you ended up with twins instead of the final child you asked for. I know I'm fucked up, awkward, and just too damned annoying and burdensome. If I could go back to that one moment I had the knife in my hand in my CCU bathroom, I would finish what I had intended. It is completely beyond me as to why you wanted me to seek help when everyone wants the insignificant flame of my existence to be extinguished.

Jessica

That (practically suicidal) note was written in my journal by my unsteady hands nearly three months before I was admitted as an eating disordered patient in Residential Treatment somewhere in Pennsylvania of mid-September 2009. I look at it now with a blank expression but feel a rush of emotions that threaten to tear down the new fragile wall of my defenses. I look at my wrist now covered with a tattoo. A tattoo placed there to hide a small and thin nearly invisible scar that continues to taunt me for unfinished business.

I have accomplished many good things in my twenty-four years, and I have had a wonderful attentive boyfriend and a group of astounding friends. A few of my college papers have been published; I've won awards. I've been here and there, partied most parties like they were my last. Done some exciting and daring things that should've put me on television or in jail. Pursued sources of excellence that for many of I have achieved.

So why the fuck am I so miserable? As far as I know, I've always been miserable, intolerant of the truth that aside from being diagnosed as Bipolar II and Eating Disorder Not Otherwise Specified with a few other *lovely gemlike* disorders, my life is worth wanting.

I can find no direct source of my misery. All I know is that I cannot rise above it. And most days, I'm just tired of fighting it.

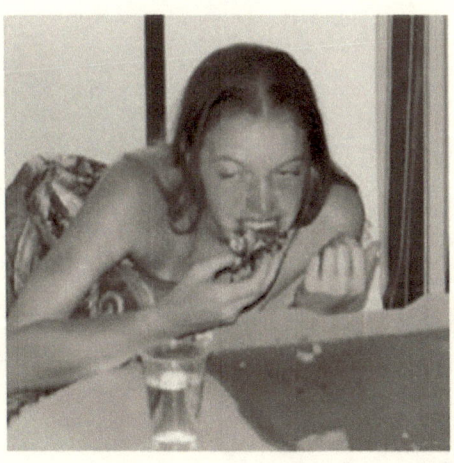

Coastal Carolina University 2006.
Age: 18
Weight: 98 lbs.
Body Mass Index (BMI): 17.9
Normal/healthy BMI for 62-inch young lady: 18.5-24.9

Take a look at this photo. Gross, right? Sunburned girl with skinny arms, scarfing down that slice of pizza as though nothing was better while wrapped up in a disgusting hotel comforter?

Disgusting.

Now let me tell you what you don't see. Having refused to eat at all the entire week before, that slice of pizza was one out of twelve slices I had in, say, about forty-five minutes. You can't see how, despite the fact I look like I am very much enjoying that delicious slice of Hawaiian pizza, I am dying to purge everything in my stomach. You can't see my slight tremble or hear my disjointed thoughts collide as my brain wastes away from starvation. The calluses on the backs of my hands from where my teeth scrape my skin are prominent, but you can't see those either. You might not even be thinking about my hair. It's only messy, right? Wrong. It's brittle from lack of nourishment, and much to my embarrassment, I now have a few gray strands.

Look back at that photo. It's more fucked-up than you realize, isn't it?

I dance to a dissonant tune, and it plays like a broken record.

Permit me to share with you the shape and size of my doom, the phony façade I have crafted, my guilt, my despair, my hesitation to grasp, and my *need* to grasp a hint of happiness and normalcy. Let me begin with the usual shy but strong introduction I have memorized for the endless string of therapists, psychiatrists, and friends I have made in Residential Treatment and group therapy:

"Hello. My name is Jessica, and I have an eating disorder."

Classification of My Disorders, Symptoms, and Consequences of My Eating Disorder

(DSM IV Diagnostic Criteria

307.50 **Eating Disorder Not Otherwise Specified**

This diagnosis includes disorders of eating that do not meet the criteria for the above two [Anorexia Nervosa and Bulimia Nervosa] eating disorder diagnoses. Examples include

1. For female patients, all of the criteria for Anorexia Nervosa are met except that the patient has regular menses.
2. All of the criteria for Anorexia Nervosa are met except that, despite significant weight loss, the patient's current weight is in the normal range.
3. All of the criteria for Bulimia Nervosa are met except that the binge eating and inappropriate compensatory mechanisms occur less than twice a week or for less than three months.
4. The patient has normal body weight and regularly uses inappropriate compensatory behavior after eating small amounts of food (e.g., self-induced vomiting after consuming two cookies).
5. The patient engages in repeatedly chewing and spitting out, but not swallowing, large amounts of food.
6. Binge-eating disorder: recurrent episodes of binge eating in the absence if regular inappropriate compensatory behavior characteristic of Bulimia Nervosa.)

I would like to add that the behaviors to each eating-disordered person is unique to them. Although I do meet the diagnostic criteria, it's not down to the *T*.

DEFINITION OF BIPOLAR II DISORDER

Bipolar II patients experience a pattern of depressive episodes (worry, disinterest in activities once enjoyed) that teeters back and forth with hypomanic episodes. There are no manic episodes or mixed episodes.

1. ("In order to receive a diagnosis of Bipolar II disorder, one must have had at least one hypomanic episode *and* at least one depressive episode within his or her lifetime. The patient must have *never* had a manic episode.")

Hypomania is a milder form of mania. These two states of mood, as well as the depressive mood, can negatively impact daily living when experiencing the episode. Symptoms include increased energy, self-esteem, talkativeness, and sex drive. Decreased level of insight, need for sleep. The patient is easily distracted and is full of racing thoughts and ideas.

DEFINITION OF CHRONIC INSOMNIA

The term *insomnia* will be used as a disorder with the following diagnostic criteria: (1) difficulty falling asleep, staying asleep, or nonrestorative sleep; (2) this difficulty is present despite adequate opportunity and circumstance to sleep; (3) this impairment in sleep is associated with daytime impairment or distress; and (4) this sleep difficulty occurs at least three times per week and has been a problem for at least one month.

A description of Body Dysmoprhic Disorder would have been included here, but there is contention about the disorder itself and the criteria that is the structure of the disorder. So just take my word for it that my "I think I look fat, most of me is misshapen, I want it to look perfect," thoughts were enough to be diagnosed as Body Dysmorphic Disordered by my first psychiatrist, who helped me realize that my body image is quite off.

I put together a list of my "symptoms" and side effects of my eating disorder. As I look at my pad of paper, I am completely shocked by the two long lists that somehow seem to come through to me more than listing them off to my medical team.

MY SYMPTOMS:

- Binging
- Purging (via exercise and vomiting)
- Downing various diet pills
- Extreme and rapid weight fluctuations
- Compulsive exercising

- Skipping meals
- Periodically checking my weight
- Calorie restricting (lowest 50 calories a day, highest 1,200)
- Frequent Web browsing for diet fads
- Searching the Web for low-calorie recipe versions of the original
- Attempted various diets
- Use of laxatives
- Buying clothes smaller than my size as motivation to lose weight
- Avoiding drinks and dinner with friends to enable calorie counting
- Developed a system of "safe" foods (foods I am comfortable eating)
- Considered liposuction and other weight loss surgeries
- Only comfortable eating foods in precise measurements
- Avoiding friends so I can purge
- Feigning illness to avoid meals
- Spending an excessive amount of time in front of mirrors to obsess about my image and weight
- Consistent thoughts of weight, image, food intake/output
- Broken up with my (now ex-) boyfriend on multiple occasions in part because I felt strange being with someone who had dissimilar eating habits than mine and because I didn't feel good enough for him
- Walked longer routes to destination in order to burn more calories
- Prefer eating alone because I feel awkward and "fat" eating in front of other people
- Feel nervous and strange with a full stomach
- Try to eat less than friends and family to engage in a silly competition with myself
- Self-mutilation cut the word "FAT" into my hip and ankle with a pocket knife as a reminder to lose weight
- Russell's Sign (calluses on knuckles and backs of hands where teeth scraped skin upon self induced purging)
- Ignored the side effects of my eating disorder because my eating disorder and body image are more important to me than the physical consequences

CONSEQUENCES OF MY EATING DISORDER

- Orthostatic hypotension and low blood pressure
- Hormonal imbalances
- Fatigue
- Dizziness
- Migraines
- Electrolyte imbalances
- High LDL ("bad" cholesterol/ low-density lipoprotein)

- Proper nutrition and vitamin and mineral deficiencies
- Fainting spells
- Fluid retention
- Decreased body temperature
- Acid reflux
- Heart burn
- Uninduced purging of undigested/partially digested foods
- Cramps/sharp pains in abdomen
- Inconsistent menstrual cycles
- Sore throat
- Deteriorated immune system
- Weakness and heaviness in lower extremities
- Cavities
- Erosion of tooth enamel resulting in translucence and weakness
- Bursting of vessels in eyes in and around eyes
- Blackouts
- Muscle cramps
- Mallory-Weiss tear (esophageal bleeding due to prolonged self-induced purging)

It is a massive wonder as to how my body isn't as damaged as it should be.

Excerpts from my journals:

March 3, 2009

Did I ever say that I detest making myself throw up? My throat hurts and my eyes are puffy. The calluses on my knuckles and the backs of my hands are now bleeding and I had to finish by shoving my toothbrush down my throat. Not one of my finest moments. I'm sure if I were in that fabled vomitorium of Roman antiquity, I'd be one classy bitch . . . but it's a shame it ain't and a shame I'm not.

I guess I'll get back to studying.

March 8, 2009

Not sure why, but I fainted three times today. I mean, I haven't been in fasting mode longer than 48 hours.

I consumed 600 calories, hardly a problem. But as I was standing in front of the fridge at 5:30 'for a snack,' my vision slacked and I collapsed. Luckily I was the only one in the house but I'm pissed that I stained my white

Free People jeans with some fucking blueberry juice. Really? REALLY? Why the FUCK is there blueberry juice in the fridge?

The second two occurred as I was running up and down the stairs. I bumped my head on the balustrade both times. Hopefully I don't have a concussion. Hopefully this headache goes away.

Maybe I should walk instead of run.

June 7, 2009

This morning I woke up, made my coffee and 'had breakfast,' already knowing I would throw it up. But when I tried, it just wouldn't come up except for fat drops of blood.

Oops.

June 11, 2009

Woke up this morning with chest pains. When I drove to Starbucks, it felt like my chest was in a vise and white stars danced in my vision for several minutes.

3:00 PM

Fainted at work. Is it because of the headache or fact I haven't eaten?

July 2, 2009

Purged day before yesterday and tonight. I feel weak, my legs are heavy, and I'm really jittery. Red spots around my eyes.

July 17, 2009

I had my physical today at one. I don't know why it was so hard to fast for the physical today because normally I fast with enthusiasm. But I woke up this morning feeling really dizzy.

The doctor told me I have orthostatic hypotension. Makes sense because whenever I move suddenly, my vision slacks or gets sparkly. He also said my blood pressure was low. To fix the 'problem' he said I should increase my salt intake. Hell, I'll do that. I fucking love salt!

Early Years and Development of My Eating Disorder

My first memory is of being in day care. It is lunchtime, and I am staring down at a gushing peanut butter and jelly sandwich. This sandwich was *literally* overflowing, and I thought I was going to be sick. Globs of sinope-colored fat and Byzantium shades of sugar tainted the white bread and plate with its promise of nourishment and its next target was *ME?*

No fucking thank you.

Mrs. Simpson warned me that I wouldn't be allowed my two chocolate chip cookies if I didn't eat the sandwich, and I would have to sit in the corner until naptime.

I looked to the freezer where she kept the cookie package. GOOD. As if I WANT the added fat! So I looked back at her and politely asked if I could please sit in the corner before naptime.

A hungry child isn't a lovable child. I was grumpy and ravenous by dinnertime, and I tore apart my parents' refrigerator when I got home. My selection? A bright red apple the exact shade of undiluted lust. I chowed down on that apple with more gusto than a kid attacking the birthday cake.

I am now eight years old. It is summer in DC. The smell of the sewage ponds would wrinkle your nostrils and singe your cilia. The atmosphere is so hot and thick with humidity that you could grab hold of it and use it as a volleyball. But my hometown is gorgeous with its riverside charm and fields of green. The various-colored skateboards and bikes. Water flickering like jewels in the light.

I don't recall what my bathing suit looked on this fateful day, but I remember a sweet and pretty twenty-something girl's bathing suit. It was a pale pink bikini to accompany her slim body and long legs. Her friend looked at her with concealed jealousy as she inquired how she stayed so thin, especially after forking down a tray of nachos. I looked down at my childlike belly with distaste then peered through the crack of the bathroom stall door to look and listen to the answer in front of me.

The girl smoothed a graceful hand over her flat stomach and spoke as though her response was Nobel prize-worthy.

"I force myself to throw up."

I heaved a sigh of relief. There it was! My answer!

Before I continue, perhaps I should mention that I was never chubby or fat, in the medical sense, especially when I was a child. BUT, somehow, I managed to believe I was. Going back to my day care years, *I wasn't yet five years old, mind you*, I was determined to lose my child belly and look like the supermodels. So it was at eight years old that I started to destroy myself.

I'm taking myself back to the evening I discovered bulimia and I am pounding the keys of my laptop in anger and embarrassment. Shame. Discomfort. Near tears for the loss of a potentially wonderful childhood.

I don't even remember what we had for dinner that night because I was so nervously excited about confining myself to the bathroom to rid my body of what I had been consuming. Now that I think about it, I was probably eating cereal because I loved it so much. It was really the only thing my parents could get me to eat.

I would stare at the back of the box, trying to solve the puzzles while absentmindedly chewing my food and only partially paying attention to my family's conversation (we usually watched TV too, but I think we talked. Perhaps I was the quietest. It's safe for me to assume. I could have asked my parents, but they had no idea I planned on publishing my quarter-life history). Then when I was finally full, I asked if I could please be excused, put my dishes in the dishwasher, and hustled to the bathroom.

Without a doubt, the deity of your choice would most certainly disapprove of what I had done to myself. It was a miserable experience, and my throat was sore, my tummy hurt, and my eyes were red and puffy. I was dehydrated and managed to look a few years older than eight. My arms and legs were weak and shaky due to the electrolyte imbalances, and I actually had to *crawl* into the bathtub for my evening wash. I think I stayed in the tub until the water cooled and my skin was wrinkly. Then I crawled out, lay on the floor to air dry myself, and forced myself to brush my teeth and guzzled a lake of water before going to bed.

Every night until my twin, Elisha, and I got separate bedrooms, we would talk and tell crazy imaginative stories until we fell asleep to the sound of our own voices. But I was too distracted that night to focus on what adventure we had planned. I was so angry but astonishingly not at myself. All my anger was reserved for that stupid pink-bikini'd girl, and I wondered if she had been playing some cruel joke on her friend. What I had done to myself was painful and felt like a chore. I wanted to slap her perfect face and prayed to God that those nachos she ate earlier would make her blow up to the size of a bovine, and she'd fucking choke on her next binge.

I was *not* going to do that to myself again, I vowed vehemently.

The next day (it was a Saturday or Sunday), I woke up early with Elisha as we usually did on the weekends to our favorite weekend breakfast of donuts (I think the last time I had a donut was before Residential Treatment). We always fought for the last plain one, but that morning, I let her have it without a fight. Then we turned on the television to watch cartoons until our parents woke and informed us it was time to finish our chores.

I was still feeling weak from the night before, and the donuts I ate hardly replaced what nutrients I lost. Stars and black fog invaded my vision every time I stood too quickly and I felt the anger rise again. Weekends were my favorite play days, and I would be damned if I allowed myself to feel weak and sick on a beautiful day.

Despite my self-damnation, I did end up going back to bed and stare listlessly at the mint green walls and borders displaying happily dancing unicorns. Their happiness bothered me, so I pulled my Precious Moments comforter over my head and curled into an angry and sick ball. I think an hour had passed when I heard my older sister, Carissa, leave the house. Nathaniel was probably engrossed in his video games, and Elisha was already out playing with our best friends. Without a doubt, my mother was out shopping, and my dad was holed up in the office as he usually was.

Feeling a bit mischievous, I crept out of bed, scratched my cat's ears, and tiptoed across the hall to the vault of treasures that was Carissa's room. I always envied Carissa because she had beautiful things, and her walls were covered with posters of the Backstreet Boys and teen heartthrobs. She had a beautiful Victorian doll with a gold crucifix standing upright in the corner of her room, and her vanity displayed figurines and jewelry boxes my fingers just itched to stroke. But that would have to wait because my mission was to collect her magazines. I made sure the coast was clear before carrying the precious loot back to my room with a goofy and moronic grin on my face.

I took her magazines because some part of my immature brain thought I would be able to unlock the secrets of the slim female form I wanted to be my own. But I ended up empty-handed as teen mags were pretty much rated G. In a fit, I not so gently returned her magazines after ripping out a picture of Brian Littrell and taping it to the inside of my closet door (if you are reading this, Carissa, sorry. I just have the hots for him and AJ).

It never crossed my mind that calorie restricting was connected to weight loss, which was a good thing, considering I was only eight years old and my concern should have been gaining healthy weight. If only I had stayed away from my mother's *People* magazines . . . perhaps I wouldn't have discovered the connection until I entered my teens. But on that otherwise fateful day, I unlocked the truth with as much enthusiasm as obtaining an award.

I hardly played sports as a child but got enough exercise exploring the marshy area of my neighborhood by way of swimming through the cotton mouth and copperhead-infested creeks, biking across town or to the pool, swimming laps instead of playing Marco Polo, bouncing on the trampoline, swinging as high as I could on the playground, climbing the big tree in my backyard . . . you get it. I was an active child, and as such, I should definitely not have limited my breakfast to a piece of fruit and foregone lunch on most days. Dinner would be my main source of sustenance; then there were days when I was utterly starving and would binge on freezer junk food or bake a pie and eat it in one sitting or hide sodas in my room just for when I needed a pick-me-up.

Family vacations or dinner outings were really the only time I allowed myself to eat properly because the foods seemed so exotic, and I was literally starving. Now that I think about it, there is a family portrait that hangs above the family room mantle that features Elisha and me sitting at our mother and father's feet. Elisha looks quite healthy and happy with her cheerful and infectious smile whereas I look too skinny with dark circles under my mischief-glinting eyes and a smile that hid the truth from my family.

The photo was taken on one of my favorite family vacations, down at my paternal grandparents' home in Brays Island, South Carolina, where they had lived in for a few years. I think it was a Christmas vacation because I remember presents and all my paternal extended family being present. My grandmother made her coveted no-bake cherry cheesecake, and I wolfed down three slices every night before coloring my Disney princesses coloring book and playing with my cousins.

What I loved most about the vacation, aside from seeing my extended family, was the convivial spirit, as though food was abundant for everyone in the world and weight was just a number. For those few days, I was a normal child, oblivious to the definitions of cholesterol, fat, weight gain, and calories. Then we went back to Maryland; I stepped on the scale and nearly had a heart attack because I had gained five pounds.

This makes me snort and roll my eyes because I'm reminiscing the time Elisha and I visited one of our aunts in Chicago. We loved visiting her because she would allow us to feed the stray kittens, play with her ferret, jump in the pool, and ogle her jewelry collection. She was funny too, and you would most certainly find Elisha and me in a heap of giggles. I don't recall how old we were, but we were young based on my short height and the fact that I nearly freaked out that I weighed forty-five pounds. All I could think about was how to avoid making cookies with my other aunt that evening.

I didn't, of course, because baking chocolate chip cookies with my mom's older sister is a past time. Sometimes the dough wouldn't even make it to the oven and Elisha, and I would be too full to eat a baked cookie. Then we would watch old movies with our aunt, sluggish and full, while repeatedly asking if Doris Day had married Rock Hudson (no, for obvious reasons). Come bedtime, Elisha and I would wait until the coast was clear so we could sneak into the kitchen for more cookies.

I'm laughing again because this reminds me of the time Nathaniel, Carissa, Elisha, and I spent the night there again, probably only a few years later, and we were so disruptive and uncaring about Carissa sleeping. Our cousin Kim had ripped open a bag of Funyuns, and instead of eating them as we intended, we stuck a few down Carissa's pajama pants and laughed, wondering what sort of anger we would receive in the morning.

Childish prank aside, these memories make me wonder why food is a regular feature in creating pastimes and traditions with family and friends. Why is the conviviality of a family feast more memory-worthy than any other part of a family get-together or vacation? Why do I associate more fondness with hazy memories of baking and cooking than, for example, the clearer memories of fishing with family down in Florida or sitting at my great grandmother's feet while listening to her talk of her childhood? I really should be able to answer this question because I graduated college with a BA in anthropology with a focus on cultural foodways. Yet the only answer I have is of personal note, and that is because I was hungry.

The Unwanted Rite of Passage, Abuse of Narcotics, and My First Lover, the Mirror

Thirteen years old and in the eighth grade. It was lunch period, and I was sitting with two friends, struggling to focus on what they were talking about. But the pain in my abdomen was completely unbearable (despite my unusually high tolerance for pain), my skin was clammy and pale, and I had my knees drawn up to my chest in an effort to drive away the cramps. Fifteen minutes passed before I finally excused myself, grabbed a bathroom pass, and discovered in the stall that I had my period.

This was a very terrifying rite of passage for me not because of the pain and presence of so much blood, but because what I had learned in health was finally happening to me. I wasn't ready for this shit, nor did I want it. I remember going to the nurse's office, bathroom pass still in hand, and asked her if she had any pads or tampons. Her eyes grew wide, and I could see a hint of a smile on her lips, and it angered me. But I pushed it aside, took the pad, and made several attempts at effectively attaching it to my underwear and then wondered if anyone could see the fucking outline.

I cried when I told my mother. and I remember her support getting on my nerves. Couldn't she tell that this was unwanted? Wasn't there any way of returning this rite of passage? WHY WASN'T ANYONE HELPING ME?

Elisha was thoroughly grossed out when I told her, but I think she was a bit jealous I had gotten it before her (Elisha is a mere two minutes older than I, but she still holds the maturity rank). I wanted to tell her she could have it because I didn't want it. My mother bought me a pack of maxi pads and tampons, and I waited until it was over.

I was so relieved when my first cycle was complete because I could fantasize that it was all a horrible nightmare. A sick and twisted prank that my body and God had played on me. But my body changed so quickly that year . . .

Training bras were replaced with new and itchy garments of torture because my own torturous chest filled out that coming summer, and my hips and waist curved out into the beginnings of a womanly shape. New jeans were bought because my once-gangly limbs could no longer fit into the pants befitting a ten-year-old boy's body, and I was now shopping at all the "cool girls" stores that Carissa frequented.

That summer, my parents had a spa house and pool installed in their backyard, and Elisha and I threw our fourteenth birthday as a pool party. It was a blast really, but I spent more time in the water and only got out when my bladder was about to explode and when it was time to cut the cake. I was too embarrassed and self-conscious about walking around in front of my friends, especially the boys, because my figure had changed so dramatically, and I looked like a manatee in my stupid flowered tankini. My big fluffy beach towel was my only comfort as I wrapped it around my short form and hid myself from view.

My four years of high school are a bit of a blur, and I'd prefer not to struggle to dig deep into those memories because those four years were a big son of a bitch. Sure, I had friends and good times, but I was also a standard nerd, a socially awkward moron (also very sarcastic . . . seriously, can't anyone understand the sarcasm?), and was picked on for it quite a bit (it didn't help that my enthusiasm for getting into a magnet school program in biotechnology only heightened my nerdiness). But these were also the years that my problems became more pronounced.

Up until high school, I had been on medication for ADHD and symptoms of depression (years later I would be diagnosed as Bipolar II), but I just stopped taking the medication as an act of rebellion. I didn't like having to take medication to control myself, and I think it took a lot of whining to my mother to convince her I didn't want to take the meds. I wonder what my life would be like now if I hadn't stopped taking the meds because my moods and attitude took a turn for the worse.

I remember being up all night some nights because I was on a high of positive and fidgety hypomanic energy. I would turn on my lamp in the middle of the night to scribble down thoughts that swam through my head, and I would do pushups and sit ups to tire myself out. Elisha would always crack open the sliding doors between our newly separated rooms and hiss at me to turn off the light, but I would ignore her and continue to sweat out my energy. *I have calories to burn here!* I remember once hissing back.

Those nights constituted perhaps only a few days of the month and any other night would be filled with depressive insomnia. I can't really remember a time my mood was balanced out when I wasn't medicated. I think I only fell asleep when too tired to function because the nightmares were too ferocious for me to face. Two things happened here, both that would continue my destructive path.

The first would be my dad taking an interest in exercise due to his back problems. Before I continue, I want to make it very clear that my father had no direct part in my eating disorder. He never pressured me to exercise and always told me I was beautiful. But with my hypomanic energy, I did use his equipment (quietly in the dead of night during my hypomanic episodes) and put together my own weight loss program.

The second would be my profound interest in sleep aids and drugs (sorry, Mommy, and Pops). It amazes me how well and functional my liver is right now because of all the pills I popped until the summer after Residential Treatment. The pills I swiped mellowed me out and brought me sleeps so deep I would have mistakenly been in a coma. Sometimes I would take them to school with me and keep them in the protective padding of my pockets and take one before math and skip out of the class to claim illness and sleep in the health center. Then I would take another after work, tell my parents I wasn't hungry for dinner, and would go to my room to sleep and shed skipped dinner pounds.

By the time I was seventeen, I weighed 120 pounds and stopped growing at sixty-two inches. A perfectly healthy weight for my height but I wasn't having *any* of that healthy nonsense. In a matter of months, I had lost the extraneous twenty pounds; thanks to one meal a day and a thirty-minute walk or jog around the neighborhood. I felt like shit, but at least I was finally skinny.

The one thing I remember most about being seventeen is walking past my dad in the foyer so I could run upstairs to my room. He looked at me with scrunched brows and asked me if I had lost weight.

"I dunno . . . I *could* have," I replied dumbly and scurried off to my room to grin in triumph and strip down to criticize my appearance in front of my long mirror.

I'm sure it's not hard for you to imagine a love-hate relationship with your mirror, but can you imagine spending forty hours at a minimum in one week just standing in front of it to analyze and criticize every inch of yourself? I would read in front of this mirror, pausing between each paragraph to look and see if I suddenly grew a few inches, lost my breasts and hips, and shed unwanted pounds. I would eat in front of this mirror in an effort to disgust myself enough to want to put my plate down and work off what amount of calories I consumed. And sometimes I would sleep in front of this mirror because it seemed friendlier than my comfortable but nightmare-inducing bed.

My Binging, Purging, and Fasting Habits

How would you define "binge"? Without firing up your search engine of preference for a definition, how would you describe "binge" in your own words? (You did look, I'm sure, because I did too.)

Of course, whatever legitimate definition you settled on is accurate, but If you were to ask me to give to you a definition of "binge," I would give you a blank empty stare that betrayed the brain of mine working in overdrive trying to figure out how I could define it in a small paragraph!

BINGING

A binging episode is unique in its own, to the episodes, and is dependent on the mood of the eating-disordered person. When you found your definition of binge, it sounded something like "indulging a behavior or pattern to an excess," right? This is true for me, of course, and more.

Binge eating is graphic and disgusting, and you know it when you give into to it, but you just can't stop yourself. You need that food in you *now*. You don't really chew. You haven't even fully swallowed the previous bite before shoving more into your mouth. Your hands and mouth are moving at a speed that would do you good at the county fair hot dog eating contest if ever you were to enter.

Then you stop, perhaps five minutes later, maybe sixty minutes later. You got crumbs on you, your shirt is stained, you shrug it off, head to the bathroom, and purge it all up so you feel clean again. The only problem (aside from the obvious fact that this is all deadly behavior?) is you don't really remember it all because these episodes are frenzied.

That's all true for me. These are my "unique" behaviors. But I have more.

During my fasting periods, the words "binge" and "excess" are shaped into a new meaning. The graphic description of what I have revealed to you is no longer. Not until I feel the frenzied need after weeks of starving myself.

I try to restrict my caloric intake to something between fifty and six hundred calories during my fasting episodes. And I start with a number as low as fifty because I know I am weak and have to take into account a certain amount of calories I will binge on in a day. Very often I am strong enough to keep it low, but if I NEED THAT 1/4 CUP SLOW CHURN VANILLA CARAMEL ICE CREAM IN ME RIGHT NOW BECAUSE I NEED TO CRUSH THESE FEELINGS WITHIN ME, I just gotta.

And it's only a one-fourth cup. Surely that doesn't constitute a binge, does it?

It does. To me, it does. Perhaps not to you or the scientific community, but to me, it is a binge, and many other eating-disordered persons would agree it is the same with themselves.

One more thing. I have often wondered if it would be safer for me to purchase only the grocery items I would absolutely need, or if it would be better to "empower" myself by adding a few "trigger/fear" foods (food items that spark a binge) to the "safe" foods (foods I feel comfortable with/foods that enable my disorder) mix.

Dunno. Neither ever helped.

FASTING

I can't remember a morning I have woken up and haven't planned my caloric intake for the day. Well . . . there was going into Residential Treatment and not being *able* to, but I did try to select the lowest-cal food items per meal. Anyway, I wake up in the morning and (after lying around in self-pity, wailing about how my body is being unfair for needing calories and disgusting for being too curvy) think about what I have in the kitchen, what I want to eat, how much of it (usually one-fourth to one-half each item I plan to eat), and which meals I prefer to have for the day. Alcohol took precedence over food too, so there was decision to be made about how many beers or diets and whiskey I planned on having.

The calorie restrictions depended (still depends, I suppose) on the current weight, how shitty/guilty I was/am feeling, and how serious I was about sticking my restrictions down to the calorie. I've joined weight loss forums, claiming I was one hundred pounds overweight, just to get the motivation and support I needed to lose what I thought needed to come off (they're really gung ho and scary motivational, these dedicated people on the forums).

Sugar-free energy drinks, pots of bold coffee (bold and black as carbonado, please), cigarettes, sugar-free gum—I think these things have known my body in my mid—to late teens to present more than solid food has. They helped me hold off on this habit of eating (though my brain was screaming at me to feed myself a big fatty rib eye with caramelized pearl onions, potatoes smothered in sour cream, chives, cheese, butter all washed down with a good microbrew IPA). I don't think I realized until this moment that the constant consumption of the aforementioned appetite suppressants would drive me crazier because it reminded me of food. The need to eat. How much I wanted to eat but couldn't.

There were only so many excuses I could make to family and friends to avoid meals, so I am sure these patterns became suspicious. Why wasn't I eating? Why was I losing weight? Teenage girl phase? Ill? Stressed? The issue was never brought to conversation until the discovery of my evening bathroom dates.

Well . . . I suppose there was one excuse. The medication I take to put me to sleep at night was one of the most effective appetite suppressants I have come across. I lost fifteen pounds in one month. Eventually, my weight plateaued. That was a valid excuse to having lost weight but not so much when I convinced myself that the appetite and nausea side effects were still present, and I still couldn't eat.

HOARDING

Whether or not my binging, purging, and fasting habits coincide, there is another habit of mine that coincides with the fasting, binging, and purging with every episode in a lapse and relapse. It is called "hoarding."

I'm certain you have heard of hoarding. How could you have not?

I hoard my calories, and this usually occurs in the evening when my stress levels are high, the house is too quiet, and when my binging and purging episodes are most likely to occur. Calorie hoarding is simple. I fast during the day, or at least nibble on low-calorie food items, and then I will save more than half my daily intake for that evening in one sitting.

Let's say I plan on 1,200 calories today. I'll eat an apple for breakfast, a super low-cal yogurt for lunch, snack on some sugar snap peas. That puts me around 200, maybe 250, calories before dinner. Come dinner (if I eat with my family), I anticipate an extra 300 calories if I don't have a salad. So let's call it 550 to be generous.

By 10:00 PM, I'll only have had 550 calories. That leaves me with 650 calories to go. Now, I'm not going to eat something with low calories but filling at the same time. Absolutely not. I'm going to eat a bunch of shit until I. AM. STUFFED. And these items will take me to 1,200. If it is a purging evening, I barf it all up, and that takes me down again.

Aside from the purging, this can cause problems. I'm not eating enough during the day, and that makes me irritable. And I'm pretty much useless, mentally and physically, when operating on such a low amount of energy. And my stomach and intestines were probably annoyed after my hoarding because now they gotta work overdrive. I guess hoarding isn't "as bad" as the binging and purging, but it's still not a healthy habit.

This is really all I can give to you on the subject of my unique habits without going on a book-long tangent, but I guess I should throw out there that purging and starving myself aren't all I know or do. I can't think of a very noteworthy activity at the top of my head to share with you, but I'm sure there is one.

March 31 2009

Next Week Plans
Water fast - April 1 and 2.
Fruit and veggie fast - April 3.
Cardio - April 4 and 5.
April 6 - fruit and veggie
April 7 - cardio and 1,200 calories
April 8 and 9 - fruit and veggie
April 10 and 11 - 1,200 cals and cardio
April 12 - Easter.

April 7, 2009

I threw up again today and guess how many calories I consume in a day? Less than 400. Seemed appropriate.

August 15, 2009

I am so disgusting. Just binged on a sugar-free pudding cup. I tried not to purge tonight, but the urge was too strong because a miscalculation of calories prompted me to do so. I would rather die than gain weight.
Remarkable how a little tiny bit of purging can make one feel so weak. My arms are shaking and I can no longer hold this pen.

Body Image

My body image really is atrocious though I am able to hide it from most people. Those who don't know me, those who are only acquainted with me, and most of those who *do* know me, I have conned with claims of loving myself (*BLECH!*). The truth is I hate *EVERYTHING* about my body. I think my boobs are misshapen, my hips and waist too wide, my upper arms too short, and my elbows too knobby. But what I *hate most* about my body are my *goddamned stupid thighs*.

I hate my thighs so much (so much so that cutting had been directed most at my thighs, as you will see soon, a photo of the word "fat" I had cut into the flesh of one offending thigh). I'm short, that's for sure, but I hate how my shortness makes my thighs look. They look somewhat "OK" when I wear heels or boots, but most of the time, I just want to hide them. I don't like how they touch at the top. I don't like how they look like upside-down Christmas trees. I might as well join a farm of fat-thighed animals because I would fit in so well! Send me back in time to live with those of the Gravettian culture because they would *worship* this horrid body of mine and *love* to use me as a model for their Venus figurines!

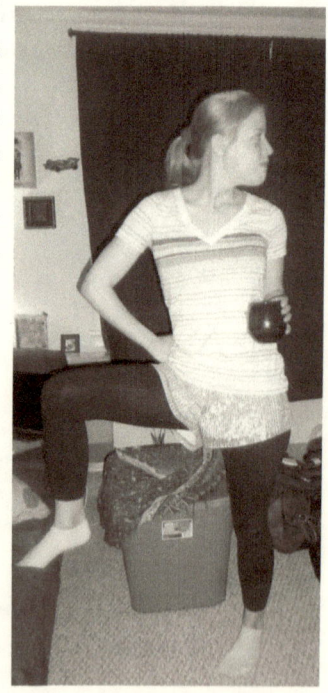

But seriously, take a look a look at these thighs. I'm 105 lbs. in this photo and MY. THIGHS. ARE. *HUGE*. And they flare into massive hips! Holy shit. My upper arms aren't small enough. And look how short they are! OMG. Why is one boob higher than the other!? My calves are too fatty too.

Shit. I'm acting like a group of teenage girls criticizing themselves in front of the mirror.

I guess you're probably thinking I was properly diagnosed with body dysmorphic disorder. You probably think that what you are seeing is a normal human female body, but what I see is all backward and upside down, and I wish that vodka sugar-free Red Bull drink in that cup was in my hand right now.

12:30 AM, May 31, 2009

I hate myself so much. My thighs touch. All I want is to disappear.

July 24, 2009

My thighs SCRAPE TOGETHER! I'M FAT. I have to lose 10 pounds before school starts.
One week until the beach.
Fat ass.

September 12, 2009
Went to a body dysmorphic disorder correction therapy session, and it was pretty intense. We did some exercises that had us asking ourselves "how can I believe 'this' is how I look?"
Fuck if I know. I'm just fucked up.

Wanting to Look Unhealthy:
Bitter for Being Unhealthy

Text Message to Residential Treatment Friend, Shauna:

> *I actually think a lot of women, even non-eating disordered, would get annoyed or angry if someone said they looked healthy. But I don't care about them. I need to express myself through my body and I don't want to look healthy. That's how I want to express myself.*

I'll break this text message down for you, as the issue and content may sound a bit confusing.

My friend Shauna and I were discussing how it really bothered us when someone says, "You look healthy," to us. It's in our nature to think this way, that healthy is bad, healthy might mean "fat," and for so long desiring to whittle away our bodies, it just fucking angers us. It's irrational, but that's not how we see it.

I have always wanted to look waifish and have a smaller cup size and thinner thighs and smaller waist. I have been called "waifish" and "haggard" when I was at my lowest weight and "skinny," "thin," and . . . *"healthy"* at my highest. Therefore, "skinny" and "thin" are associated with my "healthy" weight; therefore I consider it to be a negative association. I will still use the term "skinny" to describe what you would classify as "skinny" as my description and viewpoint could be just nonsense to you.

There's also the matter of me needing to express myself through weight loss and keeping an unhealthy appearance.

I've never been particularly good at anything in my opinion. Really. You couldn't even consider me a "jack of all trades master of none." Sure, I've done some shit somewhere in time that deserved recognition, but those were breaks from being a dumb ass. An eating disorder—*my* eating disorder—is something I excel at. Something I am *good* at. I deserve an A fucking plus from my disordered friends who are still wrapped up in the grip of their own mental turmoil.

Sadly, I have gotten that recognition, and ever sadder were the big smiles I gave for those sick twisted comments and the fiery glow I felt in the pit of my stomach. They asked me what I do in particular to keep "skinny," but I wouldn't say. Even I know that's fucked up to tell an eating-disordered person how I do it. I'm not going to be liable for that. Plus, in my opinion, that's like writing a paper for someone else or sharing your content with them. I did the research for my own damn paper, thank you, and will not be reprimanded for someone else taking the content that was *mine*. The content being my methods of "staying" skinny.

(And more importantly, I don't want to be that twenty-something lady who revealed her secret to a friend that she barfs to stay thin. I don't want a child to overhear my secret and begin that child's life's journey into hell. I would die a thousand excruciating deaths before I allowed that to happen.)

But I *need* to look unhealthy. I don't care if someone thinks I look too waifish and haggard. *Pfft,* I've only heard those said once because when I lose weight, it's all redistributed to my boobs and my stupid hips.

I've never had amenorrhea (the loss of a woman's menstrual cycle), but I used to wish I had because (1) having your vadge bleed once a month is damned annoying (*OH!* BUT I CAN'T TAKE ORAL CONTRACEPTIVES BECAUSE THE THREE BRANDS I TRIED OUTTRIED TO FUCKING KILL ME), and (2) it's another indicator of being physically unhealthy.

I've long since passed the desire to lose my stupid period because I seriously don't want my bones to go brittle. That's what happens. I would rather have bamboo sticks shoved up my nails before I develop osteopenia or osteoporosis.

Look . . . there is another reason I don't want that shit. All these physical internal issues I have, I mean. I've seriously hurt myself, and with that comes the consequences.

I tell people I don't want kids. If I changed my mind, I don't want them until my late thirties. I tell people I find kids disgusting, needy, and annoying. That description is actually true in my opinion but the real truth is—

I was born to be a mother. I honestly thought I was born just to be a mom. Despite all my issues, despite my fears of getting fat and ripped up during pregnancy, I was really born to be a mommy because children move me. They make me smile. Their enthusiasm, wonder, and innocence warm me. But then I was told that due to certain medical issues and side effects of my disorder, the chances of conceiving are pretty slim.

Tests weren't done, but the thing about me is if I'm given bad news, I don't want to look into it. Because if it ends up being true, if I'm given all the details, it will rip me apart. I would spiral downward into a relapse so deep that I would never break free of it. So I'm better off not knowing. It's better for me to convince myself that I don't want kids.

As I had been writing this bit about children, Shauna and I had talked about the subject of kids. It was quite sad really. Wistful . . . seemingly hopeless. We wondered if we would get to the point of having a garden, showing our daughters how to plant, to take care of animals.

Oh, how I wish. But even if I could have kids, I'd have to straighten my shit out first. I'm not . . . I'm not so sure I could do that.

I would like to make it very clear that I would never pass on my tendencies to any child. All these behaviors that I have developed have been kept entirely to myself. I would never make a child feel self-conscious about him—or herself, and in terms of nutrition, I would certainly try to have the child fulfill the serving sizes and food items suggested by the USDA (United States Department of Agriculture). Children are meant to be loved, not broken down.

I suppose more should be said on the subject of health. I mention later on about how stress and my eating disorder have weakened my immune system, but it deserves more explanation, and I think this is the perfect place to do so.

You eat properly to keep your immune system in tip-top shape. If you are sick, you take a break from exercising so you don't aggravate what's already been aggravated. When you get hurt or ill, you take necessary action to ensure you will recover.

I have taken none of those actions in the past, and sometimes these days, I still don't. I didn't/don't eat properly so I would/may stay thin, and that goes with the exercise too. I've never been one to take necessary action because of a high tolerance to pain and fear that anything I have done to myself would have been discovered.

But what if I had been bitten by a venomous snake or spider? In my area, although it is necessary to seek treatment, a healthy adult would survive a widow or recluse bite. But what about me? The mountain I lived on with my ex-boyfriend Grey was a playground for black widow spiders. I would see at least one a week, the hospital wasn't far but it was still a ways, and I wonder if had I been bitten, would I have survived?

What about high fevers? I am too stubborn to go anywhere (unless it feels like strep or a UTI) for treatment if I have a high fever, as will be further described in the chapter about CCU and Suicide Attempt. I get dangerously high fevers; and by not seeking treatment, I am playing with death, especially with my weakened immune system.

Of course today, what with *trying* to stick with healthier eating habits and forcing myself to see a doctor when I am ill, I'm sure my immune system is chugging along there, even if in a weakened state. But there is still the fear of what could happen if my immune system can't kick an issue on its own. It really scares me. Because I don't want to die, no matter how suicidal my thoughts may be at times.

Oh, one more thing. When someone else learns about my eating disorder and my "I think I'm fat" dialogue, almost always the reply is, "But you know you're skinny, right?"

GAH. After I say, "I think I'm fat," how could I possibly *know* that I'm "skinny?" If I did, might I not have a problem as severe as I really do? The question makes me uncomfortable more than annoyed. Because somewhere in the back of my mind, I do know I'm not fat, but I don't want to.

Self-Mutilation

I think self-mutilation deserves a section of its own though I will keep it short. I want to keep this brief and get it over with because to be honest, this chapter embitters me. I am bitter because I miss cutting myself. The feel of the blade pressing and dragging into my skin. The sting of my skin splitting. The fiery sensation of peroxide against wound. The hiss that passes through tight teeth. The brief reprieve from life and fears.

Anyway.

Did you know that an eating disorder so happens to be a form of self-mutilation? I had no idea until I was in one of my many group therapy sessions in Residential Treatment. So when I thought cutting was the only form I had engaged in, the eating disorder was the worst of it (I think eating disorder as a form of self-mutilation is bullshit because I'm not looking to harm myself with my eating disorder . . . per se). And combined . . .

All I can do is reiterate that I am a disturbed individual.

Back track ten years ago. This is important because it will infect these next eightish years of my life and with progressive frequency. When I was fourteen, I started cutting superficial slits on to my skin. Mostly my arm because I seemed to carry my stress there more than any part of my body, and the release I got from the knife was like an all-consuming drug. My mother noticed once, but I told her that my cat scratched me. I'm sure she didn't believe me, but she didn't pursue it especially since I switched to cutting my ribs to be more careful about exposure. I stopped for a very short bit when I was seventeen, but my habit came back with a vengeance at Coastal Carolina University only a few months after stopping. Cuts remained superficial as did the bottles of peroxide.

Self-mutilation was another method of releasing my feelings through another medium of discomfort (although there is hardly ever any pain). Since I couldn't talk about these feelings, the cutting seemed only natural. Like I was bloodletting a tainting and toxic disease. And I loved the sting of the knife slicing through my skin and the sting of the peroxide against the cut. I focused on the sting instead of my thoughts, and I felt better for a while.

These days, my cutting habits are rare though I do find myself wanting another tattoo (I told myself after the second I would stop there, but big surprise, I got a third on my ribs) because the needles stabbing into my skin is just . . . wonderful. Like scratching away an itch. And although startling, accidental cuts are always welcome too.

I think I'm relieved that the little scars have disappeared from my ribs, but some of them remain on my forearms. I'm ashamed about the word "fat" I have cut into my skin, and hopefully, it will go away. But it will be forever in my memory and right here.

I'm glad it's not the clearest of images.

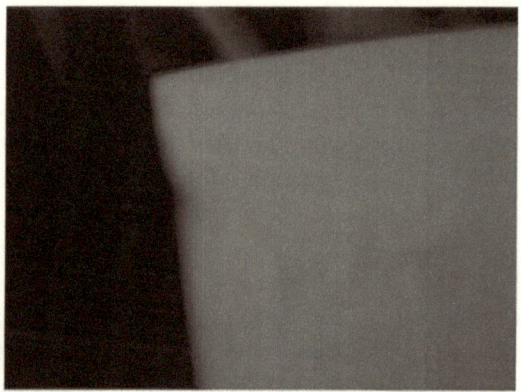

Insomnia

Sleep is very precious to me. I get little of it, but there are those rare days where I can sleep seven days straight, only waking to shower and force myself to eat a little bit of something, perhaps cereal (gotta love cereal), drink some Gatorade, and then go back to sleep. This will happen about once a year, and I wait impatiently for it like a child waiting for Christmas (or a different holiday, I suppose). The last time this happened was Christmas break, December 25, 2010-January 3, 2011).

My issues are more pronounced when the insomnia awakens from its short dormancy and overstays its welcome. Especially when my depressive episodes kick in. What a *joy* it is to have both as company because the binging, purging, symptoms that resemble PMS and the feelings of being burdensome and fat are as large as a mushroom cloud. They're like the monsters finally breaking out of my closet and crawling out from under my bed and just laugh as they push me back and forth, like bullies do.

About a week into my new job in 2012, I wouldn't take my insomnia medication because I was worried it wouldn't wear off when I needed to wake between 5:00 and 5:30 AM. I started out taking 25 mg instead of the prescribed 100 mg (though I missed the 100 mg because it caused me to lose my appetite and helped me effortlessly lose weight. I was skinny again, but I looked tired and rough around the edges). It proved hard for me to catch some sleep until the second week when I became so exhausted that I fell asleep at 7:00 PM one night. And then the next night, not being tired in the least, I absentmindedly took 50 mg. When I awoke, I was so wobbly and dizzy and still feeling the effects of the medication that I blasted some East Coast hip hop in my car, slapped my face a bunch of times, and guzzled a giant bold coffee while chewing instant coffee grounds for safe measure. I texted my mother to let her know I got to work safely. And it took two hours for the medication to wear off.

Once it wore off, I was exhausted by my efforts to stay awake and to keep my vision focused. I had two hours of downtime to kill, and instead of napping as I should have, I drank another bold cup of coffee. Then another. Maybe I added a sugar-free AMP to the mix? The point is that I was flying high on caffeine and became so jittery and my eyes so bloodshot that I could feel my heart racing. It worried me, but at least I was awake. I wrote, drew some shitty pictures, danced, checked the air pressure in my tires, checked the oil in my car (it was clumpy and low), all in the span of ninety minutes. Why did it sound like my car was revving when I put it in park? Better watch the tachometer for a couple minutes.

I wonder if I ever had this sort of energy during my hypomanic episodes.

I can't blame doctors for treating insomnia as an internal imbalance, genetic, or an effect of any disorders such as depression, bipolar disorder, anxiety, what have you. I get it. I think I believe in medical science more than I believe in God. But what I don't understand is how they and my family and my friends think that one little pill will treat chronic insomnia and so thus my bipolar II disorder, anxiety, self-mutilation, body dysmorphic disorder, and eating disorder (so many disorders!). What do they know of what insomnia—and in my case chronic insomnia—really does to *me?* Unless you are affected by any sort of insomnia, I can answer that you don't know *shit* about what it does to me. You are asked uncomfortable questions (and therefore have to dig deep into your mind for the scary and traumatic memories you have tried to repress) and all because of that sleep is further elusive.

I almost committed suicide because the lack of sleep was killing me itself. I lie awake at night and wonder if it will happen again. I wake up after two hours of struggling to sleep and then manage to exhaust myself to a couple more hours by sobbing like a little bitch because I can't clear my fucking head of any sort of depressing or suicidal thought. And even simply *telling* me to clear my head, as simply as saying, "Take the trash out," is bullshit because don't you think I may have tried that? Insomnia can destroy everything within you, emotionally and physically, and put you in a little box labeled Destroyed and Psychotic. And you begin to wonder if people actually think you are crazy if they didn't yet know.

I tried cutting back my caffeine intake and increasing my weekly dose of the dreaded exercise, but to no avail. Sleep still evaded me, and in my current episode—as I am telling you right now—the dark circles beneath my eyes have turned to black-and-purple bruises that not even the most effective correctors and concealers may hide. I had one person tell me it was okay to get help. I was baffled by his statement until he handed me a card and told me he understood spousal abuse. It was at that moment that I realized he thought I was in an abusive home or relationship. I looked like I had a black eye because I forgot to TRY to conceal and correct one eye's under eye circles! See? *See what happens when I don't get my fucking beauty sleep?* People make all sorts of wild assumptions based on what insomnia can do to your appearance.

12:30 AM, May 31, 2009

Abusing sleep aids again but I guess it's better than the drugs.
I badly want to apologize to everyone I love. At some point in my childhood I had become the abnormality; my focus on food, diet, weight,

looks . . . they are all I care about and I want my family to know I never intended for this to happen. I am not self absorbed or vain, or even trying to impress anyone. All I want is to shrink and disappear . . . to remove myself from the world and stay out of everyone's way.

I am such a burden.

I love you, Mom and Dad. I am so sorry.

I'm sorry, Elisha. I look up to you because you are so perfect, and you can never know of my failures.

I'm sorry, Grey, because you dote on someone who is a total failure. Oh God, I'm so sorry.

8:30 PM

Had a pepsid. Heartburn was persistent all day. I hope it's not a side effect of my purging. My pulse feels funny too.

January 21, 2007

Went to Boardwalk on the Beach with Sam and Kate earlier. Had fun at the aquarium and walking around. Am back in my room now and can't sleep.

I managed not to eat anything today except for a small side salad but the girl I hear in my head keeps screaming at me that it was too much. Maybe I shouldn't have added the low fat ranch dressing? I guess I'll do some sit ups.

(Three hours later) 2:00 AM

I keep hearing things outside. Tried telling myself it's just a wind tunnel or a tree but I look out my window and see nothing. Maybe it's just the pipes.

I'm going crazy. Popped some oxy but can't sleep. I am wide awake. Too scared to move.

This doesn't really have anything to do with insomnia, but it's a subject of sleep, and as this bit will be short, it seems appropriate to stick it right here rather than have a section of its own.

I imagine it was hard for Grey to sleep in the same bed as me. These nightmares of mine are terrifying enough for me to scream in my sleep, either aloud or silently, but I suppose it wasn't aloud as often as I suspect because I was never shaken awake except when I would start to whimper or say strange things. Grey often told me the indecipherable things I say in my sleep were a tad . . . strange. Scary. Perhaps seemingly demonic.

Often, I have audio-recorded myself while sleeping, just for kicks, to laugh and scratch my head in confusion about what the hell I was trying to say in my dreams. They would be silly. But they dramatically shift to the whimpers and a frantic and ruptured breathing noise that I can only assume would be my silent screaming. I do think it's strange of me to have nightmares about hell and demons, but I suppose when you make your own hell with so many disorders, it's probably not strange at all. And I'm sure it's not at all strange for me to relive a . . . a *necklace* incident either, an incident I will tell you about later on. It will be brief.

I also kick in my sleep, and I often wonder if I have ever kicked Grey. Me being so short and him being taller . . . I'd hate to think I have kicked him in tender areas. I'm not exactly sure why I kick, but I'm confident it's a common sibling thing as Elisha and Nathaniel kicked in their sleep too. At least I hope it's common. I'd be feeding my hypochondriac tendencies if I did a full search on the Web about this issue. Not sure why I'm telling you I kick. Perhaps a heads-up. Maybe just some light humor.

There's also the matter of sleep walking. Now this is quite dangerous, for me at least. Often I have found myself outside in places I don't recognize, and sometimes in the morning, I'll find a refrigerator all torn up. That part is not exactly danger to my well-being, but to my sanity . . . how much have I eaten? How long did my binging session last? Why does my throat feel sore and my neck swollen? *Shit.* I must've purged too.

These places I find myself in: I've walked around my neighborhood in my pj's and woken up by my mailbox. Or I'd be sitting at the pond. Sometimes my feet would be *in* that disgusting pond. When I attempted a postgraduate program in Canterbury, England, I found myself outside my accommodations, standing at a lamppost, rolling a cigarette between my fingers.

Most of this isn't particularly relevant, but I find it interesting, so perhaps you will too.

Normality

When I first began to slowly realize that my eating habits and feelings toward my body weren't exactly *normal*, I began to overanalyze things. What are normal eating habits and feelings toward one's body? Could non-eating-disordered persons be considered normal in this country where a Barbie body type is valued? Is it normal to care about your body shape and what goes in it? Or is it abnormal not to care? If eating disorders were more common than healthy eating habits and mind-sets (I seriously doubt that would ever happen), would it no longer be considered a "disorder"?

Psychiatrists and therapists (at least the ones who have had "the pleasure" of meeting me) really bother me in the way they fill the sessions with what I consider to be mindless chatter. They do point out that eating-disordered behaviors aren't normal (well, *duh*, why else would I be there?), but there are . . . hm . . . *certain other* habits of mine that they consider to be abnormal and not-so healthy. I talked about this "certain other" habit with Shauna, and we both agree that this is just nonsense where we are concerned.

It was what they have described as "binge and purge shopping." You can do an Internet search for a more extensive explanation, but I'll provide a basic description.

Binge and purge shopping is comparable to food binging and purging, yet the only thing you mutilate is your bank account. Another similarity is the frenzied *need* to shop, to numb away the torturous feelings that have clawed their way into the binge-and-purge person's mind. There is the "What have I done?" feeling when they look at all their shopping bags and their shiny but frowning credit card. Is there only a hazy recollection of the shopping episode? I'm not sure. Never felt the need to binge and purge via shopping when all I needed was food and a toilet to empty my stomach into. Or a treadmill to burn off a fraction of those calories I binged on.

I have heard some of the teens and other women in one of my many hated sessions in Residential Treatment explain that they have used shopping as a numbing outlet, so I guess it's a real diagnosable thing even if it isn't in the DSM IV (I'm not sure . . . maybe it is. Don't care). But I wanted to rip my hair out when the therapists and psychiatrists suggested *I* could be diagnosed as a binge-and-purge shopper.

For fuck's sake . . . women LIKE TO SHOP EVEN ON BAD DAYS BECAUSE IT IS NORMAL AND RELAXING TO FIND A NEW PAIR OF SHOES OR HANDBAG OR WHATEVER THEY FANCY, without putting a dent in their bank account. Or maybe it does put a dent in there. If I put a dent in there, it's because I've had my eye on an item, wanted it, bought it. But I would patiently wait for the next paycheck to refill my coffers that wouldn't all be spent on shopping (I got bills to pay, a gas tank to fill, prescriptions to be refilled, hair dye to be bought, and a chunk of change saved for emergency purchases . . . like getting the fuck far away from here to start over). Furthermore, shopping is a distraction from episodes of lapse and relapse. It sets me straight for however long I browse through the shops.

I'm certain it's normal for women *and* men to feel self-conscious. To feel judged in certain aspects (sexual performance, intelligence, physical appearance, et cetera). This is normal. However, eating-disordered persons take this to a higher level. You would believe we are at an apex of paranoia. This certainly holds true for me. I feel watched and constantly judged (probably another reason I am a socially awkward moron).

Wearing a bikini is very stressful for me because I don't know if eyes are on me in appreciation or disgust. The scars have faded from my ribs, but there is still the matter of cellulite, stretch marks, and uneven tan lines and even stupid spider veins (is it the leg crossing?). And this has never been a "trigger" but more as shock and suspicion if some guy tells me I have a great body (LIARS!). I have always thought they reached the bottom of the barrel if resorting to flirt with me is an act of desperation for sex, attention, or validation, or even worse . . . they are playing a cruel joke on me.

I've never been one to effectively articulate what I try to say, so what I try to say ends up going on in a ramble, sometimes completely off point, forgotten, or even worse: I stammer because the words come out faster than I can finish the sentence in my thoughts. This makes me feel very unintelligent, and I can't help but wonder if anyone ever thought, *My God, please stop with this butchering of the English language.* And sometimes I talk too much or not enough.

Eating in front of people is another dilemma for me. What if what I order grosses someone out? Do they judge me for ordering an item too largely portioned, too fatty, or not befitting the stereotypes of what a woman should eat? What if the way I chew is annoying? I especially freak out if I eat in front of a guy I'm not too familiar with because what if he perceives me and only me as a gluttonous pig?

I'm paranoid that others judge me by the way I fold my laundry. The way I dance. Exercise. Sometimes walk with a limp. The way I hide my eyes behind dark sunglasses and pull a hoodie tight over my head when my ears and scalp get cold and my eyes hurt on sunny and sometimes cloudy days (this is a pretty suspicious look though, so it's probably why I get stared at, but I must hide myself from those who judge me for being eating disordered).

Am I judged for the way I take meticulous care in cleaning the leaves of my orchids with lemon juice?

Judged for liking snakes and spiders?

I feel judged for the way my hair frizzes even after applying a healthy dose of antifrizz and thermal active control and a good flat ironing. And judged when I don't wear makeup (rare). I feel judged for having a period (because God forbid a woman's uterus sheds its lining to stay healthy!).

In truth, those examples are silly in comparison to what I will say next . . .

I give up on wondering if everyone judges me for being eating disordered. Either I am or I am not. Judge me if you want on this one. Say it to my face. I *do* care, but the cat's out of the bag. There will never come a time when I am no longer a pariah. I'm being honest about everything I have tried to convey already. So why would I bother trying to fix this bigger picture before the aforementioned ways I feel judged?

The point I'm trying to make is, I'm just abnormal.

I'm sorry. I keep leading you in circles. I have admitted to you, and it remains the truth, that I am so miserable. Why else would I want to kill myself? But . . . I want to make it clear that it takes only small things to delight me for periods at a time, and it is these things that I think help me through my days. I can become so mesmerized and taken by small things that you would just mistake me as slow-witted.

Take for example how natural light causes a pigeon's blood ruby to sparkle and send a kaleidoscope of color dancing on white walls. Imagine the tickling sensation of deliciously cool water lapping at your ankles and soft sand swirling around your feet like a calm whirlpool. Remember your first amazing kiss and all that followed. Breathe in the aroma of coffee beans and the scent of sap and pine in the winter. Giggle when your dog is miffed he can't get to the groundhog beneath your shed and laugh outright when you see the goofy expression on his face when you splash him with pool water. Smile when a baby's tiny hand clutches your finger.

I love listening to music on long drives (Portishead and MF Doom). I enjoy watching sports (I'm a Caps and Skins fan, and pretty bloodthirsty when it comes to UFC. I'd like to make a shoutout to Urijah Faber). God save your soul if you interrupt me from reading because reading is a reason for living (you are so screwed if you interrupt me during my *The Gargoyle* read). And I *love* collecting makeup, jewelry (my collection is either too expensive or classy for me to wear regularly, but I still waste my money on it), and shoes (from heels to chucks, to shit kickers).

These things and more grant me happiness and the illusion of normalcy.

A Few Things to Clear Up: Being a Pariah

I have been called selfish, childish, immature, stupid, disgusting, and have been branded as a pariah for having an eating disorder (good God, what would they say if I told those wrong few about my self-mutilating tendencies and suicide attempt?). To these judgmental few who have labeled me as such, fuck you and go to hell. I will see you there, of course, but "I hope you are damned" is the point I am making. I wish I could have said those words to those few who have said those hurtful words, but I was too flabbergasted to even respond with a simper and a tear.

Let me clear this shit up. I have tried for many years to think of the ways in which I could be selfish for being Eating Disorder Not Otherwise Specified. There are no reasons I can come up with other than an outrageous assumption that through my bulimic tendencies, I am wasting food that starving people are desperate for. I guess it holds some merit, but was I thinking of those starving people as I crammed my mouth full of food and purged it up in frenzy? No. Especially at eight years old? *NO.*

Another person had the gall to tell me I was selfish for wanting to die a slow death while so many others lose their lives, and I quote this man, "Especially those who have died on/during 9/11."

At first I thought, *Wait, what? That's random. And how is this food related'* But then I thought, how *dare* he put one of the worst tragedies of American history on my conscience? I was *thirteen years old* when the towers went down, the Pentagon took a beating, and my fellow citizens lost their lives. I mourned the loss of so many, and I was scared for *months* just living so close to the Pentagon. I remember to this day the smoke burning the blue sky and the worry that spread through the country like an epidemic. My eating disorder came about *years* before this tragedy, and had I been able *to predict* this tragedy, I would have either been labeled a terrorist (or hopefully a hero for preventing the loss of so many). But I'm not Nostradamus with his spooky quatrains.

Childish and immature are not descriptions of which I would apply to an eating disordered person. We don't physically flail our arms and belt out wails that only a baby screaming into a megaphone could accomplish. Immature? Not at all. Sure, some of us could be immature in general, but eating disorders are not built on a foundation of immaturity. They are grounded by self-hatred, inner turmoil, traumatic events, and something I can only describe as a burning desire to be dead and alive at once.

Stupid? Me? I shrug to that one. Of course it is stupid of me to mutilate my body inside and out when I know it can kill me. But it is hard to let that sink in when all you can think when you wake in the morning is *I'm still alive. Good. I can do this again, today. I'm not going to die. I won't die. I'll be very careful about this. Oh God, please don't let me die just yet. Thanks be to you for keeping me alive! I can do this. I am in control of myself. It's not like I'm committing suicide!*

Disgusting? Of course it's disgusting. I'm barfing away my pain and, in the process, destroying my insides the exact moment the undigested food comes back up. I am whittling my body away to nothing where one would just tense up and cringe if they ever saw me at my lowest weight. *I draw blood* when I can't binge and purge as an outlet.

Listen: I am a pretty blunt person but tactful unless piss drunk. So can we exercise the same tact, and please be a bit quieter when you don't use your library voice *in* the library while mentioning to your friend that my too-slender form beneath small but baggy clothes is disgusting. I wouldn't be so offended if it wasn't your intent for me to hear.

I *have* been branded a pariah. I have mentioned to a few close friends at St. Mary's College of Maryland that I was going into Residential Treatment, and I'm sure I shouldn't have mentioned it to one of them because she is one of the biggest blabbermouths I know. St. Mary's has a small student body, and the school itself is its own little bubble. I hung out with all sorts of cliques there, and sure enough, news spread like wildfire. My only consolation was knowing that there were still bunches of people there who didn't know me. But that was until a friend of a friend would point me out to others as we would walk by each other.

If I entered the cafeteria and picked out the healthy items to fulfill my stupid USDA nutritional guidelines, some idiot would whisper, "OMG. Those are *carrots* with *light* dressing on them! Is that all she is going to eat?" right before I would go get a slice of the nasty pizza. If I were to go to a Townhouse Greens party or hang out in the Crescents (both upperclassmen accommodations), someone would slyly tag along to the bathroom with me (claiming they would hold my hair back if I felt sick from too much tequila. I knew their real intentions). Or they would just stand outside the door and listen closely to hear if I was jamming my fingers down my throat. And sometimes I did it to give them a show because they angered me so much for being annoying snoops.

I have even had friends who began ignoring me because "it's kinda . . . *uncomfortable* to be seen with you while you are in this . . . *condition.*"

Hmph. What a waste of time. For them and for me.

Oh, another thing about this pariah business. After my month-long stay in Residential Treatment, I decided to pop on campus for a visit with my friends for what the students call Hallowgreens. As I was getting my two-day parking pass (though you don't need one for Hallowgreens), the girl handing over the pass asked me why I took the semester off and I blurted "medical leave." She looked at me and asked, "You didn't try to kill yourself here, did you? Because we can't allow students on campus who have tried to do so."

"No," I said, acting confused.

Not exactly. Oh, do you want a specific date? Well . . . I'm here to party, so . . . bye.

She found out a few weeks later, I think, and our encounters were strained; and I could feel the discomfort emanating from her as though she thought that just by looking at me, she would contract some disease.

It was never my intention to commit myself to becoming a pariah. Really. It's hard to ignore the stares, the gossiping, the distancing, and sometimes the very strained efforts to make me feel welcomed and comfortable in a particular setting where eating is involved even though no one really wants to deal with the binging, purging, and fasting they think will occur at that event.

I'm damned tired of it. I can't stop anyone from judging me, nor can I unmake myself a pariah. Issues such as these are hard to ignore, and I understand that. But that doesn't mean I don't want them to be ignored and forgiven.

I want to be accepted into a circle free of any disturbance. But of course I would disturb that circle by being disturbed, so it's all wishful thinking, isn't it?

Alone

I've always felt a pressing need to be alone. As a teenager, my skin would crawl as I sat through my classes (although I enjoyed all except the war between math and me), and I would frequently go to the bathroom and breathe and wait for these mentally shattering episodes to pass. The bitch in my head would cackle like the witch she is and remind me she would be back every class period. Her presence was like a cloud of never-ending smoke in my head. A deafening waterfall. She swallows me whole every day. During my hypomanic phases, I would brew a pot of coffee (though I would already be wide awake) because as ridiculous as it may seem, she was my muse. She helped me stay thin, and she helped me develop my passion for books and creative writing.

When I would go home from school, I would crawl into what I refer to as "the bat cave" being my bedroom. If I went into the basement and one of my sisters would join me, I would flash back to the bat cave and force myself to do four hundred push-ups to regain my sanity, as ironic as that sounds. I would ignore supper every chance I could as during the dinner conversations, there was just so much talking.

Soon came the time I earned my learner's permit, and my mother and I would snap at each other like dogs fighting for just one scrap of meat because I was either driving too fast or being aggressive (soon I would balance caution and aggression when needed). My time to receive my license was as slow as a sloth-slug hybrid, and the day I did earn it was the only rite of passage I ever cared for. I felt free and happily alone just driving around my hometown, to the good side and the bad and down to the river where I would find my perfect little beach and dip my toes into the icky water. I ignored the lighters, empty bottles of Sudafed, and the blackened spoons that littered the area.

I would gaze across the water and wave to *Virginia* and watch as the ferry slowly chugged along while I felt my life was the same: slowly chugging along. Then feeling so alone (which is what I always wanted. of course, because the imminent doom of anyone not accepting my need to please crushed my soul), I would run down the hiking path with my jeans chafing my legs and the flipping of gravel in my sandals causing my sore feet to bleed. With my arms to the sky, I would spin until I could no longer stand, and then I wait until my buckling legs could move me back to my car.

I went on a walk with my mother down to the neighborhood creek, a cool summer day in September 2012, and she told me my need to be alone possibly stems from her own family. As in for lack of a better term, genetic. I suppose that is true despite the fun family gatherings in Chicago. My maternal grandfather is a quiet man, always preferring to watch television over spending time with us, but my aunts and uncles loved to sit and gossip with us. Despite my maternal family living so close to each other in Aurora, Batavia, and Joliet, I don't think they visit each other much and just enjoyed seeing each other once in a while. But I could be wrong. I never asked.

I love to read, and I am never without my Kindle Fire and two paperbacks in my purse. I have only two favorites and they are *The Gargoyle*, written by Andrew Davidson, and *My Name is Red*, by Orhan Pamuk. Otherwise, I read historical and contemporary romances, classics, suspense, medical thrillers—you name it.

Grey used to say I was more invested in my relationship with books than my relationship with him. He was right of course, and it is quite sad how I readily agree. Books just . . . well, they . . . hm. How can I put this?

My heart aches and my appetite is weakened when I don't have the flavor of the day in my hands. Sight and sound cease to "exist" as I invest my attention to the flow of words into sentences, into story on pages that feel soft and crinkly and comforting. I imagine myself as the heroine, the villain, and I create the scenery in my head (sometimes even draw it out) and sometimes imagine a few twists in the plot.

And when I am done with the book, I feel sad and alone and just have to put another in my hands and continue the marathon of reading to counteract the sadness and loneliness. It would have been more loving of me (and *SANE*) to turn to Grey to counteract the flow of emotions, but I didn't. And a frosty brittle air would possess the room when Grey noticed I was reading rather than paying attention to him after his long hours at work, and I would snap at him to let me figure out what happened next in my novel.

But in my lonely little world that I have created for myself were characters that accepted me into theirs. My priorities are a tad off, don't you think? Preferring to find company with books rather than the man I loved?

I suppose I just feel safer with friendly imaginary characters rather than those who love me. And safer from my friends who say behind my back that I'm the girl guys would like to fuck but never take home to the parents. Safer from rude and creepy dates who violate me with bold and disgusting words.

Just safer from reality, really.

Grey

How can I begin to describe such a wonderful man that was my boyfriend of six years? Grey is just . . . he's *Grey.* I'm not trying to make him out to be a god but . . . he *IS* and *WILL* remain the most wonderful person that I know because he's *him.*

He's tall and handsome, funny, witty, and playful. My parents liked him immediately even though he is nearly nine years older than me. I have to say that Grey became a big part of my life, and six years later, I don't remember what life was like without him even though our relationship status has changed.

I first met Grey only a month before I was to head down to Conway/Myrtle Beach to attend Coastal Carolina University as a first year student. We saw each other four times before then, and astonishingly, I couldn't wait for each interlude that would defy my entire being of craving solitude. It scared me of course, because how, at eighteen, could I change thirteen years (I'm sure I started fearing the company of others at age five, and I'm not sure why the company of others scares me) of this pressing need to be alone?

I knew that I was different, but I always thought that everyone craved alone time more than being with others despite the supposed enjoyment of companionship. But I desperately wanted Grey to ask me to be his girlfriend, and when he did, my heart sang. And then he added that it would be until I was headed off, and then we would see where it would head. He couldn't see my hurt, but I said, "Of course. I understand." But there it was, that impending doom that finally crushed my soul and the reminder that no one needed me or even cared to want me. How silly is that? He asked me to be his girlfriend, and all I felt was that I broke my cardinal rule of being alone. My heart is just safer when I am alone.

Grey was headed back to college too to complete his degree in business, part-time so he could continue his job as an auto mechanic. I suspect today that and the six-hour distance between us was why he said we would see what would become of our relationship. It makes sense, doesn't it? It didn't make sense to me at the time.

To my selfish delight, Grey visited once the first month and then progressively twice to three times a month. The rise in the frequency of his visits was because of my need for his company and due to my so-called friends ditching me because apparently they thought partying was more important than doing homework and I didn't have my priorities straight by choosing to do the latter more often.

Again, no one wanted me or needed me. I despised those valley-girl bitches and the douche bag frat boys I hung out with, not because they ditched me, but because, again, I broke my rule of being alone. It was the selfish depressing me who manipulated Grey to make more visits, and only a couple months after, he dropped out of school. He told me he was going to anyway, but I didn't believe him. If you are reading this, Grey, I am so very sorry. Your studies could have given you a promising career, and I blew it for you. Do you secretly hate me for that?

Come the much awaited end of my first year. I was elated to spend more time with Grey. I would drive to his place in Fairfax to spend a minimal amount of nighttime with him before I drive home because of that damnable Provisional license that gave me a stupid curfew. But the hour-long drives to and from Fairfax gave me my needed solitude. I would go to work and listen to my iPod to avoid speaking to the other interns turned employees, despite my enjoyment of their wit, sarcasm, and humor. Not to brag, but I think my boss actually allowed me to listen to music because I got the job done. They did too, but I was quieter. It was repetitive work, so how could one fail?

Once I enrolled in community college and improved my grades with honors courses and the Renaissance Scholars honors program that took place late at night, the lust for solitude slowly crept back. It was my first lover, and my betrayal to it stabbed me in the gut and slowly twisted the knife. I became jittery again; the ants crawling beneath my skin returned, and I began to shut down again right before Grey's eyes.

I never expressed my feelings to Grey, not only because I feared he would discover my decayed emotions and lifestyle, but because my family never really talked with each other, and it became ingrained in me. My mother and father were always so busy, Carissa never really wanted to spend time with her brother and sisters, and despite being raised by Nathaniel, he was off on his own getting into trouble. Elisha tried to get me out of the bat cave and hang out with her friends, but she never succeeded until college.

Anyway, I'm rambling. Back to school and Grey. Once I started to improve my grades, the compliments and praise started to roll in. I react poorly to compliments, sympathy, empathy—you name it. When someone says thank you, I'm sorry, congratulations!—and my most hated, "You can do it!"—I visibly cringe and am sometimes hit by a wave of nausea. For a good show, I put on a fake smile and then go to some empty room and calm down. I'm not used to upbeat attitudes, and I guess it stems from needing to be alone, and I'm just not used to those attitudes.

Negativity is what I respond best to because I can reply, in like, with sarcasm that completely flies over the negative commenter's head. Not Grey though. He had similar sarcasm, and soon it began to scare me that we had things in common despite my batty behaviors and his ability to cope with anything thrown his way (aside from those times I put our relationship on hold). I think he could sense that I was drifting away back into my need of aloneness, and he tried really hard to keep me from going back to that dark hole. He's not much of a people person either, and it made us kindred spirits, however much we needed each other.

I never wanted to cuddle because it induced foreign feelings (and also my stomach fat made me feel self-conscious when it pressed against his body) of what love is and a calming sensation that scared the shit out of me. I've never been calm and collected, and it was a hard burden to kick.

"You can try to be happy," Grey would say to me softly, for he knew the darkest recesses of my mind. I would grumble, "I'm happy being *un*happy."

You may not understand it, but it's all I have ever known. Therapists tried to instill it in me and even the annoying group therapy sessions in Residential Treatment. I hated how some of the other girls could completely transform their behaviors. It was grating to my sense of being, and it became more of a nuisance since I couldn't hide away in the room provided for me. But there were some girls there who were completely hopeless individuals, just like me, and I disliked them too. I talk to a few of them to this day but only once in a while. Social networking sites are amazing for my friendships with them and my need to be alone because I don't have to see them directly. Talking to them is a cruel reminder that I am just one fucked-up puppy. Or maybe . . . I don't know. Fuck it. Fuck holding it in. I miss them. I need to see them this very instant. I would be very happy with a reunion.

I did have many happy moments with Grey despite my preference for unhappiness. He made me laugh, and we talked hours on end about our own views of religion (I am Catholic whereas one wouldn't know Grey believed in a god or not unless they asked). He reminded me that I'm beautiful (I cringed just now because of the memory of the compliments), and we would kiss because I liked his kisses. I dragged him to the mall or the outlets and laughed at his miserable expressions, and he smiled before complaining about the smell of Bath and Body Works and the instant assault of Hollister fragrances upon your sense of smell. He made me giggle when he said those things, but I would haughtily reply, "I *like* Hollister." Then I would raise my chin and pretend to be offended. I used to enjoy our hikes in the snow and having summer picnics together, but that was before five years into our relationship that I shut down completely, again.

Four times I have broken up with Grey because I just *couldn't* be the girl he loves. How could anyone love a grotesque being like me? He deserved better. I wanted him to hate me because it would be easier for him to move on. But I always crawled back to him and begged for his forgiveness because his love for me was enticing no matter how much I want to be left alone. But to be honest, I hated how much I needed him. So much so that sometimes it made me cry when I had alone time.

I will admit that I was the villainous girlfriend. Unlike Grey, I am impatient, hotheaded and short tempered, crazy beyond repair, and a selfish cow. I started all of our fights, and God love Grey, he put up with it and I can't say how. It is truly disappointing that this man, with all his love to give, had ended up with the lost cause that is me.

No, but seriously, *why* did he insist that I was perfect for him? July 25, 2012, marked the sixth anniversary that we met. Now please don't sneer. I understand that most believe only married couples should celebrate such Hallmark holidays like that, but I think that is bullshit. Perhaps a two-week or sixth-month anniversary would seem to push the limit, but six years is a long time. Nor have we ever planned on marrying each other so soon, so why not start on the day we fell in love?

I'm rambling again. On Sunday, September 16, 2012, Grey and I had a nasty fight that lasted from 1:00 AM to about 4:30 AM. It started out with me seeing a strange light flashing on the ceiling, and he told me I was just seeing things. *"I am* not *seeing things!"* I hissed. *"Watch the fucking ceiling between the bureau and the pole!"* This went on for about ten minutes until he finally saw it and determined that it was the smoke detector. It needed new batteries.

How the hell was I to know it was the detector and needed new batteries? Since I have lived in his home, I have never seen the blasted thing flash on the ceiling because we tended to cover every source of light in the room before we went to bed. Pitch-black is how I love it and hate it.

"Just calm down, Jessica," Grey said tiredly. "It's not your nightmares come to haunt you."

Imagine a volcano eruption. That was me. The anger inside me blew to the sky, and I screamed at him things such as "You don't understand me," to which he responded, "Yes, I do." I won't get further into detail about what was said, but I will say I threw a horrible temper tantrum.

The day before, I had packed my things to take back to Maryland because I now live there to be closer to work. I had about three heavy boxes and two duffels to carry, and I declared I wanted to go home that instant.

Because I am a brat, I shifted the argument to three weeks before when I told Grey I was going to live with my parents again. He was pretty angry and upset about that and said, "We're through if you do that. Find a job closer. This would move our relationship backward if you go home."

"What have I been doing since fucking December?" I roared. *"I can't find one out here and, as I have said for the past fucking month, I hate it on this mountain, the gravel is destroying my car and God forbid, when it snows, I'm fucked. I hate the cabin fever of this place. And I was relieved when you suggested we would break up when I told you I was moving out!"*

I instantly regretted those final words even though I knew I would break up with him and this time for good. It wasn't until the previous week that I gave up trying to find out why I fell out of love with him. And he needs someone who would return the showers of love he gave and not emotionally and physically pull away from him anytime he needed her (remember . . . I hate needing someone).

It finally sunk into Grey's head, what I was saying. I was breaking up with him again. He shook his head as though what I said was all in his head, but then he started to cry. I hate seeing him cry. I hate breaking his heart.

It really sucked, and it still sucks. You can't break up with someone you loved for six years and not feel insanely depressed about it. Unless you're a cold-hearted bitch or bastard.

But I hated the highs and lows of our relationship. He was always so happy and calm, and that grated on me. I would pick fights with him so he would be on the same level of unease as me, and hopefully have him hate me enough to break up with me.

It was 3:30 AM, and we were both stressed out and chain smoking to reduce those stress levels. We were speaking more calmly now, but I still wanted to go home. It seemed awkward to sleep in the same bed with the man I had just broken up with. However, I had forgotten that all lanes on I-495 were freaking closed as usual, and that was my only route home, so I had to stay.

It's awkward talking to him every day and not telling each other I love you before either one of us went to bed. I miss asking, "Did you set your alarms?" He would smile. Yes. To which I would reply, "All seven million of them?" (He really did have a ridiculous amount of alarms set on his phone, and it was hard for me to sleep through them though he slept like he was in hibernation for the winter). In the morning, I would mumble, "Don't forget your phone and wallet. Have a nice day." Then I would roll over and sleep until the insomnia medication wore off.

Sometimes I think Grey slipped away from me as though he'd finally had second thoughts about dating me. I even wonder at times if he'd been seeing someone else and because I was too scared to ask, I regularly joked, "How is your Russian bride?" It hurt to have these thoughts when he'd been so caring and attentive and tried to pull at least one hug from me at night, any sort of return of affection. He doesn't know it, but while he slept, I reached out to touch him, to remind myself he was still there, and that I am still alive. Sometimes I got out of bed, sat at the desk to chain smoke, and stared out the windows into the darkness, wishing he were in love with someone else, wishing I was that someone else, and most of all, wishing I could wake up and be a child again where I could start all over.

For a long while, I desperately tried to figure out why I fell out of love with this loving, supportive man, but once I moved back to Maryland for my job I knew it wouldn't work out. Sometimes I cry because I wasted so much of his time. I ask him if he hates me, he says no; but if I were to enter a relationship with other people, things would change. You must understand how this statement affected me. We had history together and to just know that we will have different romantic paths will or may inevitably separate us for good.

April 8, 2009

Poor Grey. He seems worried about my weight fluctuations.

April 18, 2009

Anyway, last night I couldn't stop jabbering to Grey about how FAT I AM and WHAT A PIG I AM for eating a small brownie. I am so weak for wanting it. How is he attracted to me? I'm short and fat.

Usually when I "jabbered" to Grey, this is how it went: I'll be standing in front of the mirror with a grimace on my face, turning this way and that way, making sure the ridges and contours of my ribs are still visible, making sure my thighs don't touch, making sure my upper arms don't look healthy.

"Grey . . ."

"You're thin!" he'd say in an annoyed tone. He just knew what I wanted to hear if I'm standing in front of that mirror.

I would ignore him and ask, "Am I fat?"

"No, Jessica," he would say tiredly.

"Liar," I'd mumble in return.

I know he wanted to say that this old is song and dance to it was getting old. He once threatened to remove the mirror because "it's not healthy how you use it to undermine yourself, Jessica." I threw a hissy fit, more like a parade of fear, and the only way to shut me up was for him to take back the threat.

May 1, 2009

I came home today (last day of regularly scheduled classes) because Grey was sick and I wanted to help him get better. I also bought him orange juice and rice krispie treats because they seem to be his favorite sick room food. Anyway, when I set the stuff down, I stood in front of the mirror and went through the routine. He watched the whole time as I plucked at my fat thighs and stomach. Finally, I asked him what he was staring at.

"I'm just trying to understand you." He said nonchalantly. "How can a beautiful girl like you think she's fat?"

I hate this statement so much because if I were beautiful, I would be skinny. But I ignored him because I knew if I answered, it would precipitate an argument.

Then he tossed me a box of chocolate.

He KNEW I swore off foods that turn me into a slovenly pig and now I'm a bitch for not wanting the present.

"But you LIKE chocolate." He snapped.

"It makes me FAT!" I spat.

"You are SKINNY, Jessica!" He practically shouted. But he took the box back and tossed it across the room as though it contained a rhumba of angry rattlesnakes.

When I went into Residential Treatment, I had a dream that my therapist noticed that I stuck to my journals as a method of staying grounded in my eating disorder, and in this dream, I was told I wasn't allowed to write in them unless for my literature track or to write self-reflective letters to read aloud to a counselor that I had to meet with fifteen minutes every day. I was extremely angry that they considered my journals contraband (restricted items), and I wasn't allowed to have them back until I left. But it was during a session with Maria, my therapist, when she read that last passage to me and I was overcome with waves of guilt, shame, and pettiness.

She asked me, "How does this sound to you?"

I didn't want to reply with what she called my "astute intellect," in our real sessions (puh-lease), but she threatened to extend our session if I continued to hide behind a wall.

"I sound angry at Grey for not encouraging my disorder."

Maria nodded and stared at me with her hawklike eyes that I knew meant "continue."

"And perhaps it's silly of me to think I can lose twenty pounds in an unhealthy manner and not have a problem?" I suggested in a helpful mutter.

Maria nodded. "You're in the right place," she said.

"I want my journals back," I blurted.

"It's not healthy how you use them, Jessica."

"But I can't not write!" I cried. "I want to write a book."

Maria arched an inquisitive brow.

"You can read my entries. Just please let me have my journal. I'm going mad without pens and paper!" I pleaded.

Maria sighed and handed me a new journal.

"Thank you," I said in clear relief while clutching the notebook to my chest. "I was damned close to writing on the walls."

Maria cracked a smile.

Only in dreams do I actually seem to open up to people. I didn't tell Maria about this dream, for fear of actually losing my journals, and for fear that it might help me

pave my way to recovery. I never told Grey about this dream either because as you know by now, apologies aren't my forte, nor could I ever allow him to understand my feelings.

This dream also reminded me how I really do depend on my journals to keep me grounded in my eating disorder.

Grey kindly allowed me to include a favorite photo of us in this section. It doesn't do much for his anonymity, but it does warm my heart.

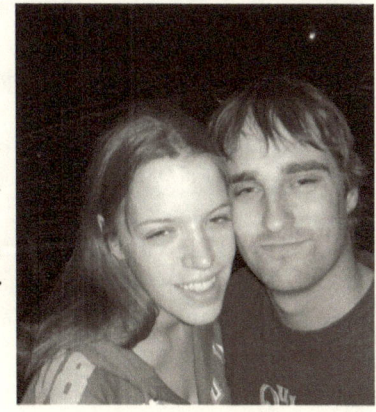

Recovery, Recovered, Triggers

Dreams. Daydreaming. Hopes and dreams.

(Bear with me here.)

Fluffy white clouds. A cool warm mist caressing your face.

(I'll make a point soon.)

That one piece of artwork that captures your attention in a museum, separating you from it by a felt rope and bullet-proof glass.

(OK. Here it comes.)

You see these things. Feel them for the briefest moment, a peaceful emotion. Look at them with such longing that you know it will weave its way through your mind like a beautiful gold thread.

All of this is bullshit, I tell you. Extreme bullshit. None of this calming shit can be grasped or even touched (except perhaps the mist, but that's beside the point). *You can't ever hold this shit that you so desire to have.* And don't even *try* to think you can. It's just something to look at. You let it taunt you.

What I am getting at is this term that the doctors called "recovered." It makes me roll my eyes, jiggle my knees in irritation in their offices when they say, "You can do it!" And I just want to bash my head into a wall whenever I *think* of the word and its meaning. Hell, I'm still on that dark swampy path of *recovery,* and every day is a trial. I think "recovered" is a poorly disguised myth the doctors try to knock into your brain to get you out of rehab as soon as possible to make way for the next batch of disordered persons.

Of course there could be a lucky few, perhaps a lucky lot of my fellow disordered friends and acquaintances who have reached that state, but I never have. Perhaps I'm being too rude about this subject, but on a personal note, I have tried—and failed. Maybe I'm not strong enough (I've hardly been one to feel defeated or give up even though my "Fuck! It's the end of the world!" attitude would seem to suggest otherwise to those who don't know me) because this shit is the hardest task I've ever faced. I tell you from experience that I've had those couple months in increments where I'm soaring through the sky and ask myself why have I ever done these horrible things to myself, but then some bad day shits on you and then you go falling back into that gutter. These are called lapses and relapses. I've experienced both in the few years that I've left Residential Treatment and even before that.

However, as you may have assumed, I am a walking contradiction. I may be extremely annoyed by the subject of "recovery," but that doesn't mean I don't want to be "recovered." After so many years of being tangled up in this mess of me, Residential Treatment gave me a glimmer of hope of what sanity and happiness could be. If I wasn't so focused on my ridiculous theory of "If I give up my eating disorder I will be fat," perhaps my views on recovery and "recovered" would be different. I admit that I should have invested more of my energy and attention into what I really went into Residential Treatment for. I was politely asked by my family to get help; I agreed, and I wasted their time.

I honestly do want to "get better." but it's hard to completely let go of what you know so well. Eating Disorder Not Otherwise Specified was my first love. A love-hate relationship of course, but still a first love who sticks around when I decide I want it back.

I have called my path to recovery "a dark swampy path." I have mentioned I'd rather not be happy because happiness eventually betrays you, and I mentioned how I could only imagine what a "glimmer of what happiness could be." I attempted to commit suicide because I was so unhappy, yet I also mentioned early on that "my life is worth living." Therefore, amidst these dark moments of my life, I have experienced happiness; though now I didn't realize that unfamiliar feeling that is something similar to the fear of feeling out of control when I am completely wasted drunk to the point of hugging the toilet in sickness.

I have often wondered if maybe I have had these flying high moments of happiness due to hypomanic episodes. But they just do not match up with how I would describe what I feel and experience during my few hypomanic episodes. These feelings I experienced . . . they *felt* almost as tangible as what I previously described as bullshit. So why am I leading you around in circles, telling you one thing is bullshit while claiming I have actually experienced them for brief moments at a time? I will tell you why, to reiterate and confirm that previous statement.

During these moments of bliss, feeling healthy, promising myself to recover, eating happily without fear, looking in the mirror with appreciation—although usually unfamiliar with these feelings, I *want* them. I *NEED* them. I commit myself to them more than anything I have ever committed myself to, and I truly believe that these thoughts would last forever. But then something would change those thoughts. It could have been caused by a bad day or, confusingly, just a malfunctioning switch in my thoughts that occurred out of the blue in a random moment while experiencing feelings of will and pride. I would feel that beautiful gold thread quickly turn into a poisonous snake's tongue and tail flickering and coiling itself deeper in me and that's when the heavyweight of doom returns.

Cold sweats. Rapid pacing. Falling to my knees while clutching my pounding skull and covering my ears as though I could protect my thoughts from the inevitable. Sometimes, I hear myself groan "No!" and "Stop!" and feel the betrayal of pitying hot tears drop to my fingers. It doesn't matter where I am. I find a place to hide and detox myself from whatever I'm feeling. It works for a little bit, but then I give up and give in to what I know best.

I'll give you a few ideas of what triggers us back into our old habits.

I think it's a rarity being triggered by each other when we call up and say, "*Hey girl* . . . um . . . I'm having these *thoughts* . . ." though they have the potential to do so when discussing these thoughts. In my opinion, that happening would fall under a different category of jealousy or working in cahoots (example: "Oh my gosh, I better starve and purge myself because I'll be so jel if I'm not as skinny as her," or "Hey, you want to starve or purge or both? Let's do it together!"), and I've never experienced that before entering and leaving Residential Treatment.

THE TRIGGERS OF A LAPSE AND/OR RELAPSE

- Stress from work, school; breakups; loss of a friend or family member; monetary troubles; hostility in friendships, relationship, and families.
- Imbalances in hormones and neurotransmitters (natural or medication related)
- Harsh words or judgment made by friends, families, or strangers (example: "You're ugly," "You're fat," "You're stupid," "You're not trying hard enough"—I've had the first, third, and fourth directed at me)
- Just one bad day
- Insomnia
- Conduits of media such as television, magazines, the radio (though it is a rarity for me to be affected by images and words related to thinness and eating disorders)
- A horrified glance in the mirror at a new wrinkle, stretch mark, or cellulite-ridden area on an already created wasteland of a body (self-mutilated, I should say) that you firmly believe will be less distressing if you lost a few more pounds (which, ironically, *made* some of those wrinkles, stretch marks, and cellulite in the first place, "but it doesn't matter because I'll be thinner")
- Putting on an old pair of jeans that are too tight or, interestingly enough, too loose, and you ponder the idea of how many more sizes you could drop (my first successful experiment with this was at eighteen years of age where my chest expanded even further and hips grew wider . . . but a pair of jeans I had purchased at fifteen years old hung loose around my thighs and waist. I promise that this is not bragging)
- Appetite-suppressing medication

These are only a few examples of the triggers that throw me into a lapse or relapse. I know for a fact a few of the above examples have slapped the pressure of lapsing and relapsing on my friends. It is not uncommon for me to receive a Facebook or text message from one of them asking to talk . . . to spill the reasons of why they have yet again collapsed. In fact, I get very worried if one of them doesn't text me or message me via Facebook because it makes me paranoid that one of my emaciated or internally destroyed friends has landed herself in the hospital or the bottom of a cold grave. I worry about that for myself too.

CCU and Suicide Attempt

I managed to drop to ninety-eight pounds before going off to Coastal Carolina University, and this was the one and only time Grey had *never* seen me whittle away before he knew the extent of my problems. Problems that didn't begin and end with an eating disorder.

Coastal Carolina University was an eight—to nine-hour drive from my home in Maryland and about six hours from Fairfax, Virginia, where Grey had lived when we first met. I vaguely remember my parents warning me that I would be homesick, but I honestly thought I could deal with it, knowing Carissa was a few hours away at school in North Carolina. Elisha had gone to school in Erie, Pennsylvania, and I desperately missed her; and years later, I recall my mother telling me it was kind of stupid to have chosen a school so far from my sister and best friend. But I was enchanted and feeling a bit smug for leaving home to pretend I was an adult at a beach school.

The first month was a blast. I made a lot of new friends, went to the beach often to swim in a skimpy bikini or read on the hot polluted sand, and would meander in the marine science lab with the poor dead sharks that had been pulled from the ocean nets. But my happiness took a dramatic shift when I began to miss Grey and my family and the beautiful landscape of my hometown.

I started to gain weight too; "thanks" to healthier eating habits and um . . . alcohol. My suite mate and I started to go to spin classes and dance classes together to stay in shape until it got ugly. I think it was Halloween (but *of course* it would happen on my favorite Hallmark holiday) when she called me a "pussy" for not wanting to go to a spin class that day, and I remember thinking to myself, *What the fuck? How am I a pussy for not wanting to go to a fucking spin class? Bikes suck, anyway, and you can wander your ass over there yourself if you're feeling so bored and fat. You're the fucking pussy for not wanting to go alone.* Not-so-pleasant words were exchanged, and I went outside to call Grey to let out some steam.

Since then, my suite mate and I smoothed things over, but our friendship faded. If I were to search for her on Facebook right now and "add" her as a friend, I'm sure she would ignore the request. But anyway, I immediately closed up because her true side became more pronounced after that, and so had my own. I was sarcastic and bitchy again and more so after my asshole friends wanted out.

Perhaps if I hadn't closed up, I might not have hated CCU, but I began to resent the school because shortly after my fight with my suite mate, I lost other friends. Why? Homework and class came before fun and partying, and these so-called friends didn't seem to like that one bit, so they immediately dropped me from their social circle. In a fit of hurt and anger, I immediately and harshly labeled the school as a gathering for the superficial bimbos and douche bags. (Anyone reading this who went to CCU, I apologize for having thought so.)

I remember Thanksgiving perfectly that year because I was running a very high fever (on the flight home), and I remember crying like a little bitch to my parents until I was dehydrated because I wanted to come home. But the question, "Do you really want to give up right now?" seemed to lend me the belief that my supportive parents didn't care. They are very caring, but because my anguish masked all rational thought, I didn't realize they had asked only because they knew I would hate myself for giving up. I wasn't exactly a perfectionist growing up, not like Elisha, but I certainly cared enough about my grades and school to hate myself if I failed any class or course (other than math). They knew that.

Back to CCU I went, took the finals, and went home for my month-long Christmas vacation. During the day, I worked at the biotechnology company I worked for as an intern in high school, and in the evening, Grey would either have dinner with my family and me, or I would drive back to Fairfax where I felt safe from the world and my destructive nature. And I ate and ate some more, drank and drank some more—all until I could no longer fit into my size 0 jeans and had to break out my size 4s. Break ended too soon, and my parents drove me back to CCU (a good thing I didn't have my car because my road rage is very ugly in well-developed areas) where they took me to lunch before settling me in again.

They told me they were proud of me for making the decision to stay another semester, and I cried in my room because I wanted to cut myself, but how could I do that without my roommates noticing; and crying seemed like an okay outlet to get rid of my stupid feelings.

That week, I had a falling out with my roommate Kate because of conflicting sleep schedules (insomnia and a roommate rolling in around 5:00 AM do not mix). The day of the falling out, I moved down the hall into a quad suite where her twin sister, Sam, lived (who eventually became my best friend at CCU), and I was presented with my own lovely room.

P.S. Kate: I hope you enjoyed your new roommate if you found her. Have you found the massive-hand-sized huntsman spider I put in the room? Oh, don't worry if she got snarky with you rolling in around 5:00 AM and finally bit you. Her bite is completely harmless.

I can't decide if having my own room was better for my health or not because my insomnia came back worse than ever, and I possibly only had eight to sixteen hours of sleep in total per week. Not even my sleep aids helped; either because I was building a tolerance to them, or my stress was too overpowering. There would be nights where I would call Grey at 3:00 AM, crying, because I couldn't sleep or because I was hearing spooky things. Anything that creaked in the night, I attributed to my dreams finally coming to haunt me. But what haunted me most was the voice in my head screaming that I was fat and worthless.

About a month later, I have had it with my weight gain. I put together a plan (I wanted to do this the *healthy* way and not restrict although that endeavor just died a day after trying it out, so now there was some purging here and there and a lot of unhealthy calorie restricting to 500-1,100 per day) and would work out six days a week and began to avoid dinner with friends and completely shut everyone out. I would only hang out with Sam and my other suite mates, two of whom would go to the gym with me or walk on the track field where we made fun of one girl running with her ratty-ass thong sticking out of her pants. Both suite mates were taller than me, and I gave myself shin splints just trying to keep up with them.

While attending CCU, the constant stress and lack of sleep had me developing colds or other illnesses every other week. I remember doing laundry with a painfully high fever and one nice guy ordered me to sit down while he went to get me water and a thermometer. I remember giggling to myself because this hot guy wanted to play doctor with me, but I hightailed right out of the laundry room of course, knowing very well I belonged in a hospital with that fever but not wanting to miss my afternoon class.

My suite mates also noticed that I was making myself sicker by still exercising while sick, and Sam even went as far as hiding my scale. I handled it like it was a joke, but inside I was very livid. That was *MY* fucking scale, and I *needed* that scale because how else was I going to tell if I lost weight? The number was as important to me as looking skinny. With disapproval and frustration clear on her face, she reluctantly returned my scale, and I released a sigh of relief.

That night, while sweating out my fever and coughing up a lung, I wrote in my journal after one incident that sometimes I wish I had finished. The date will not be included.

> Talked to my dad and he chastised me for exercising while sick. I wanted to call him a hypocrite but fighting with my dad is like engaging in war.
>
> Took my temperature after I got off the phone with him and I'm running a 104 degree fever. Took a cold shower and fever reducers but I feel weak and this pen is so heavy. Laying in bed naked and sweating holes through my sheets. Lied to Grey by telling him I was feeling better.

Later . . .

Stifling the sobs as it is 3 am and I don't want my suitemates to hear me. I did something awful and I hate myself but I wish I finished it because this stress and insomnia are driving me to madness!

I have a peroxide soaked bandage wrapped around my wrist and I don't even remember going into the bathroom for the knife. I think the bleeding is subsiding but there is so much of it. SO MUCH OF IT. I should go to the hospital but I don't want to be kicked out of school and I need to go back to the bathroom and make sure there isn't blood on the knife or counter or floors.

The next day . . .

I was able to get some sleep last night and my fever went down but I still feel like shit. I'm going to skip my classes and get much needed rest and will skip exercise today and move it to Sunday.

I remember now what happened. I was lying in bed, wide awake, focusing on the white noise of my TV to drown out the voice in my head, telling me I'm fat and worthless. I remember getting up, pulling on a t shirt and briefs and listlessly pacing my small room as though that was the only way to get rid of the voice. But I found myself in the bathroom. That industrial college bathroom with the white walls and cold tiles beneath my feet and cheap mirror with my sick and very tired reflection staring back at me. I wasn't surprised to see my t shirt already sweat soaked.

My eyes fell on the dish rack filled with cheap ceramic plates and bowls amidst cheap metal silverware and a lone wood handled steak knife. I picked up that sharp serrated knife, took it to my wrist, and sliced. But God help me, the moment I saw the blood, I hesitated. Fuck my life, I hesitated. After years of self mutilation, I FUCKING HESITATED. Years later when I tell whomever about this incident, they will probably call it bravery or the will to live but it's all bullshit. Stop with the pep talks. I hesitated because I didn't want to die a fat ass.

I missed a few drops of blood on the countertop . . . hope my suitemates didn't see them. Guess I'll wear long sleeves to hide this.

I ended up going to my World Cultures class because it was my favorite, but I periodically got up to hide in the bathroom as I coughed myself into suffocating fits (and blood into the sink). After about sixty minutes of the ninety-minute class, I stayed in the bathroom and waited until everyone had left before I could apologize to the professor. She had looked at me sternly and asked, "Shouldn't you be in the hospital?"

I looked away, and she handed me a name and number. It was her own doctor's name and number, and she wanted me to give her a call if I wasn't better and still too stubborn to go to the hospital or poor excuse of a health center. I thanked her, pocketed the name and number, and posted it on my bulletin board where it was soon forgotten.

May was my last month at CCU, and I completed my first year, passed all of my classes and stayed at 102 pounds. I was skinny again, much to my relief, but . . . couldn't I just drop two pounds? My parents took me out to dinner my last night in South Carolina, to a favorite surf and turf. They congratulated me and told me how proud they were of me for toughing out the year and that I was strong and brave. I awkwardly thanked them (*cringe*) and proceeded to stuff myself on carbs and expensive seafood, key lime pie (one of my and my dad's favorites), and later a few beers that I managed to flirt out of a guy at the hotel. Grey and his brother taught me to be a beer snob, but I couldn't wait to shotgun all six of those Natty Bohs.

The next morning, a bit hung over and cursing my low tolerance, I stepped on the scale that I packed in my duffel bag and nearly shit a brick. All the food I ate the night before was still sitting in my stomach, and the number that flashed at me was 108—*108!* I could hardly fit in a morning run because my parents and I were planning on leaving within the hour, and my dad had already finished using the gym. I decided I wouldn't eat much that day.

Returning Home, the Escalation of My Eating Disorder, Therapy, "Reminder of a Necklace Incident"

It is now summer of 2007, and I am happy to be back at the lab, working with my previous coworkers. We picked up where we left off, joking around, talking about the new guy because he was really creepy, and reminisced about our high school days where we had interned at the very same company. But one thing had changed. Because I was eating regularly (but of food befitting a herbivorous baby land mammal), I was too scared to join them out for lunch as I used to because I never knew where we were going and that didn't leave me much room for counting calories. In order to count them, I had to bring my own lunch to work and would savor the crap out of the ridiculously small portion in the conference room, waiting for everyone to leave because I felt weird and felt like I was being watched while I ate. It all sounds a bit ridiculous, but anything goes if you're pining to stay in those size 0s.

Every day after work, I would immediately hop on the treadmill and make use of my dad's awesome weight system and sets and shove my mother's healthy dinners into my face. And I still managed to be hungry an hour later. I would always freak out though, wondering if I ate too much of the high-protein dinners, so I would do leg calisthenics on my bedroom floor or in the shower while trying to focus on a book or blaring some Portishead or Taylor Dayne to not bore myself into stopping. I spent most evenings with Grey, and we would make salads or something else only befitting a rabbit. I assumed he thought I was only trying to be healthy, but the day I told him I was being checked into Residential Treatment, he told me he figured I had problems.

I had a lot of fun that summer, enjoying being at home again, spending time with Grey, using the pool again, seeing high school friends, going on mini vacations. My parents took Elisha and me to Twinsburg, Ohio, for our last Twinsfest vacation together, and while not as fun as it was when we were kids, I miss that particular vacation because it was the last time Elisha and I were together longer than a couple weeks here and there.

What I didn't like about that summer were all the visits to the dentist. I never feared the dentist when I was growing up, but I must've been to the dentist six times that summer because all but one tooth had cavities in them and the enamel had taken a beating (I assure you, I'm a meticulous toothbrusher and flosser so this can only be attributed to the purging). I assured the dentist that I brushed my teeth morning lunch, and night; flossed in the evening; and used mouthwash. But what I didn't tell her that purging was a way of life for me. This had been going on full rush and apparently with enough frequency to bore holes into my teeth and erode the enamel.

The day after we got back from Twinsburg, I had an appointment to have my wisdom teeth pulled and a canine that was causing some problems (perhaps I should have kept those braces). I wanted to be that heroic fool who stayed awake during the procedure, but the pompous doctor, after being very graphic with the talk of blood gushing and pressure of the tools, I opted to go under anesthesia (again, I have an unusually high tolerance for pain, but the doc swayed my decision). You would think that after years of self-mutilation and having handled shark guts and unborn shark pups, I would be able to handle gushing blood, but when he said "pressure," I thought I was going to barf and *not* on my own volition.

The procedure was an hour, and I woke up feeling fuzzy and more than a bit nauseated. I looked like a wild boar with dried blood crusted around my lips and cotton buds in my cheeks, but I applaud myself for having waited to get home to confine myself to the bathroom to throw up.

The thing about me and purging is both simple and complex. I don't get that gleeful feeling when I feel sick like so many of my other eating-disordered friends who use actual illness as an excuse to avoid food—because it's *my* barf. I and *only I* get to tell that stomach of mine when it will be emptied, and God help it if it decides to cast itself up. The feeling of nausea, as many of you know, is not pleasant. Neither is the sparkly vision, dizziness, and heavyweight feeling in my extremities after self-induced purging, but it's better than the nausea.

I took off work that week because I looked like a chipmunk with my swollen jaw, and I stayed in bed all day because I felt sick to my stomach. The saltwater solution I gargled to cleanse my teeth wasn't a big help either as I felt the bile rise in my throat with every swish of my mouth. I lost five pounds that week (thank God) and a lot of free time because I had regular visits to the dentist to fill the cavities and have a bridge capped over the empty space where my disruptive canine had been.

September came fast, and I attended my local community college for the second year of my college career (and for those who judge, community college is every bit as enriching and educational as any four-year institution), and I rediscovered my passion for learning (nerd alert) and changed my major from marine sciences to anthropology, a subject that had been a passion of mine since my parents took Elisha and me to a symposium on the Valley of the Kings when we were young. I took several honors-level courses and enrolled in the Renaissance Scholars program that was aimed for students who wished to excel.

I was also back in therapy, and that was the first worst and best decision of my life because it paved way for the discovery of my problems.

Dr. Carlotta was a lovely and sweet woman whose office and home was about fifteen minutes from my parent's place. Our sessions were held on Thursdays, and I remember the first day I met her. It was an Indian summer day, and I sat huddled in a big leather armchair, trying to remain warm in my skinny jeans and a hoodie that I probably swiped from Grey.

"It's not cold in here, Jessica. Are you cold?" she asked softly.

I pulled the cuffs of my sleeves over my hands and shrank further into the heat of the chair. "I'm just naturally cold," I murmured in reply.

She pursed her lips together and scribbled on her pad. Then she asked, "Are your hands cold too, or are you hiding something?"

How perceptive. Yes, I was hiding the faint scar on my wrist and the bluish tint of my fingernails. But I told her my hands were cold.

"Tell me why you are here."

I hated introductions. Hated getting into the past. I already told her over the phone what my issues were. "My parents want me back in therapy."

"But *why* are you here?" she repeated.

I also hate the questions that therapists and psychiatrists ask. They confuse me. Why can't they please be direct? Are they asking for a simple answer, or am I supposed to follow up with some dream I had that makes me feel the way I do?

"Because I hate my body, and I'm depressed, and they think something is wrong with me," I blurted in a rude tone.

Dr. Carlotta smiled as though we had made a breakthrough. "Do *you* think something is wrong with you?"

Oh, brother.

"I mean . . . I guess. I'm sad all the time for no reason, and I think I'm fat and ugly," I muttered.

This went on for a few sessions until Dr. Carlotta's smiles faded into delicate concern. Apparently, I was in need of desperate help, and she didn't have any expertise with adults with my issues. I expected my parents to ask me to find a new doctor, but to my surprise and relief, they didn't say much on the matter. I was only a little offended and hurt but mostly glad because I didn't want to be put on pills that would straighten me out and potentially help me believe I didn't need to lose weight. I was 105 lbs that semester.

Grey had expressed more concern, but because I get defensive and hotheaded so easily, he backed off. I'm sure I yelled at him to drop it.

The school year was pretty uneventful aside from my binging and purging, compulsive exercising around midnight, and habitual abuse of painkillers I collected from frequent hospital visits. Oh, there might have been a few academic awards here and there, but this isn't a memoir about my achievements.

Near the end of the year, my advisor and I looked at other four-year institutions and a summer internship at the Holocaust Museum in Washington DC. We settled on St. Mary's College of Maryland, a charming liberal arts public honors college in Southern Maryland nestled on the St. Mary's River.

"I know the dean" she said with a mischievous smile on her face. I applied but had been wait-listed, which turned out to be a real fucking bummer for me because *not once* had my applications been previously rejected or wait-listed. Sure, I wasn't going to apply to Harvard or Yale, but I thought my chances at getting in without a bat of an eye would be pretty good. This set up more self-hatred and destruction, and I felt suffocated in Maryland, again. I told my advisor that although generous and appealing, the Holocaust Museum internship wasn't in my best interests, and when I told her about three history and anthropology summer abroad programs in Galway, Limerick, and Dublin, we immediately got to the paperwork.

Convincing my parents to send me to Ireland for the summer wasn't hard. They knew that I always wanted to travel to Ireland, knew that this was a great academic opportunity, and for all I knew, was a good chance to get rid of me for a few months. Grey wasn't too happy about it, but he showed support for my enthusiasm.

All three schools accepted me into their programs, and I settled on Dublin City University because it had the longest program and would be taking us on academic field trips to the western counties (and much to my excitement, Inis Mor) and Northern Ireland. Plus, the campus was only a fifteen-minute bus ride to the city center and an-hour walk (which I found out I preferred. Go figure). The program began in late May, and I absolutely could not wait to go! I worked until it was time to leave. and I managed to lose a few more pounds before leaving.

I was a fucking mess at Dulles International. Saying good-bye to Grey for a few months was rough, and more than once I hopped over the felt rope of the security line, pacing back and forth, now wondering if I could manage to keep my cool while away. I sobbed when I finally said good-bye to Grey, sat next to a total bitch on the plane who whined about sitting next to the window (I would have given her the aisle seat, but I was having my period, and how would she really like it if I hopped over her during the flight to periodically change tampons? I wouldn't have cared about that one bit but . . . no. I paid for this seat, so fuck off), and avoided the iffy in flight meals not because they looked vile, but because I thought I could shed another pound.

The plane flew into Heathrow (my most hated airport next to O'Hare and De Gaulle). and I had a couple hours to kill before my flight into Dublin. I remember walking around the boutiques and sniffing various perfumes that reminded me of my younger years, sitting in my mother's master bathroom, watching her beautify herself for a work-related event or a date night with my father. My mother always wore the best perfumes and high-end cosmetics, and her hair was never out of place. She reminded me of a modern-day Grace Kelly, something I knew I could never achieve.

After ordering an Americano (which the barista happened to water down. I hate, hate, HATE weak coffee—it needs to be bold and strong enough to gnaw at steel),

I went to the gate, got on the cramped plane, chatted with a nice Irish lady and her husband, and met with the program leader once I got off. There were three other girls waiting, all the epitome of beauty and sophistication, and I immediately shied away because I'm such a gauche dunce. But they were nice and funny, and one of them turned out to be my roommate, and we bonded over the creepy girl who would wander into our suite to ask where I was and what I was doing.

When we got to the campus, I was expecting the usual dorm ordeal, but we were actually placed in a hotel-like dorm with beds already made, silverware and plates already in the kitchen, and a TV in the common area. There was also a balcony with sad and dying plants that I managed to bring back to life.

I think there were four of us in that suite, and we went to a small pub for dinner then finally succumbed to jet lag and slept late the next morning before classes. In total, there were about thirty American students and only one guy who, with two of my roommates, ended up being one of the greatest friends I've ever made.

The program was *awesome.* I enjoyed going to the classes but had trouble staying awake because our professors' accents tended to lull me to sleep. Three to four days a week we had classes, and it was likely that our main professor, Dan, would cancel a day or two and send us out into the city center or even challenge us to travel farther out in the country to immerse ourselves in the culture. My friends and I did so with pleasure and travelled to nearly every county in Ireland, and I soon discovered a fondness for Bushmills, Paddy's, and Jameson. On more than one occasion did we go to St. James's Gate to take a tour of the Guinness Storehouse, and God help you if you ever say the G (Guinness) word at the Jameson distillery. Whiskey practically flowed through my veins during my few months' stay in Ireland, and I think I may have abused it a bit. I'm sure my liver was happy I wasn't abusing sleep aids and drugs on this academic trip. Sleep was, once again, elusive.

With the drinking came a lot of late-night binging, and by the end of the program, I had gained more weight. Walking from campus to the city center and a lot of hiking through Wicklow, Inis Mor, and up and down Croagh Patrick had given definition to my legs, but it sure as hell didn't combat the amount of calories I was consuming. I headed back to America feeling sad and fat. But first, a few wrong paths in Heathrow led me to miss my flight back to Dulles, and I had to wait four hours until the next.

I walked around the terminal looking at souvenirs and cosmetics before purchasing a gossip magazine and coffee laden with sugar and calories. I definitely needed the girl time with the sugar and gossip because I was completely drained of all mental faculties. But before I could flip open the magazine and take a sip, this disturbingly hot guy was staring at me while his two skinny girlfriends talked about a flacon of perfume they had just purchased.

I quickly looked away and wondered if he what he saw was a fat ass about to make wild love to her sugary coffee. But when the two girls got up and left to go to the bathroom, the guy got up and took a seat next to me. With an awkward expression on my face and my lips still wrapped around the straw (because I wanted to drink it, dammit!), I looked up at him. This guy was seriously good-looking and looked ready go out and enjoy the day while my face was tear-stained (not because I missed my flight, but because I had gained weight), my hair pulled back into a messy high ponytail, and body swathed in CCU basketball shorts (men's medium . . . I like them baggy), a teal CCU sweater, and silver trainers that didn't match anything about my hideous outfit.

I looked like a hot mess, and he radiated male beauty. Tall, slightly mussed sandy blond hair, blue eyes the exact shade of periwinkle moonstones, tanned—I've always avoided the seriously good-looking guys because they (not purposely) made me feel self-conscious about my own appearance. Really. It takes me between two and three hours to make myself look only pretty*ish*, and in my opinion, they roll out of bed already glorious.

"Uh, hi," I said awkwardly. I'm sure I sounded like Kermit the Frog because my voice was hoarse from crying and purging.

Turns out he wanted to buy me dinner and drinks before the flight. It boosted what minimal confidence I had to have such a hot guy asking to buy me dinner and drinks. I wanted to giggle because he was such a hunky sweet-talker with a light sense of humor, but I declined and informed him I was in a relationship and would so happen be meeting my boyfriend at Dulles. The guy shrugged and went back to his seat, and to my luck, he sat a few seats away from me on the plane, but his staring became quite uncomfortable. It gave me cold sweats. I became paranoid.

The last guy who stared at me like that with such creepy and frequent intensity tried to choke me, or play a game by choking me, with a favorite necklace I had been wearing. Which is why I freak out when someone tries to touch my neck. I *really* freak out when someone reaches for my neck in any manner. I freaked out when Grey tried to joke about my adversity to anything touching my neck and the considerable discomfort about it by mockingly reaching for it, leaving me in suspense because I didn't know if he was going to touch my neck or not.

I didn't know the guy. Didn't even recognize him. It was dark outside. I went home, tried to shut it out, and pretend it was just a game. A few weeks later, I felt guilty about not reporting it. This guy could have done some serious physical damage to me (I hope killing me wasn't his intention, or else I'd have some other girl's death on my conscience) and succeeded with the psychological damage. I should have gone to the police. But I had been drinking. Maybe had something else flowing through my veins, like syrup.

I should have told someone. But I felt like I would be more of an outcast and needy if I did.

I never told Grey or my parents. They would have asked too many questions, and this was almost a decade ago. But I won't go into further detail about that experience. I won't. Because I feel ashamed. So don't ask. I shudder to think what would have happened if I hadn't broken the chain of my favorite necklace. I never told anyone about this before now, nor will I when they ask me why I would ramble about it here and not in therapy. I won't even say where this happened.

My point is . . . all I'm saying is that guy at Heathrow was giving creepy stares, and I'm also miffed that I usually attract the creepy dudes. And because I was fucking scared the entire flight back to Dulles and it had me sick to my stomach in the gross bathroom. But at least that helped me shed a little bit of unwanted weight.

None of this was the hottie's fault but, *sheesh* . . . be a little more covert with the stares, buddy.

Anyway.

Let me be clear that I wasn't the most attentive girlfriend while away. I admit it. Words Grey never heard directly from my lips and will only hear it as he reads this. I called him every day and chatted online with him every day, but I think the most we talked in a week was twenty minutes total.

When I saw him in baggage claim, I was overcome by hot waves of tears and wanted to beg for his forgiveness. But the first words out my mouth were, "I got fat." Clearly, my priorities aren't in the right order.

Grey looked lean and handsome whereas I gained weight. It really wasn't fair, in my honest opinion.

When we got to his car, he kissed me and gave me two belated birthday CDs and assured me that while I gained weight, I wasn't fat.

Weren't all boyfriends supposed to say that?

I called my mom from the airport to let her know I landed and would first be going to Grey's house before coming home so she might not want to wait up for me. But she did, and when she woke up from her sleep on the sofa, she said, "Oh, thank God. When you said you got fat, I literally expected you to be fat."

You might be thinking what an odd thing for a mother to say to her daughter, but she didn't sound relieved at all, nor would she have even told me I was fat if I was. I think she was saying it mostly for my benefit, more commenting on my lack of perception, and that weight didn't matter.

You can't really see how I have gained weight in this photo because of the billowy hoodie (and also because you have never met me?), but it's shown in my face and my thighs. Those aren't the smallest my thighs have been, and I am completely grossed out by this photo. My face is the width of a Thanksgiving ham, and my thighs like logs.

Anyway.

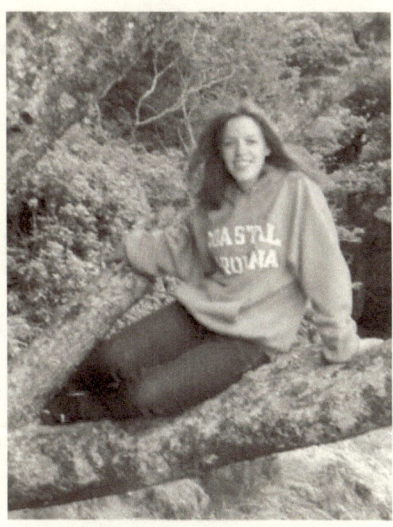

Photo taken in Connemara 2008

The next evening, my parents asked me to come into the living room, and I thought to myself, *Oh, God, who died now?* Instead I asked, "What did I do?"

It turns out that my paternal grandfather had died that summer of a heart attack while sleeping. "While you and your friends took your trip to Scotland," my mother said softly. "We wanted to tell you, but there wouldn't have been time to fly you out to California in time for the funeral and have you back in Ireland in time before classes started again."

I was in complete and utter shock, so much so that the tears were backed up. It was when my father said, "I miss my dad" and began to cry that the tears finally fell. I had never seen my father cry before, and it was very overwhelming and discomforting for me to see.

"How is Julie?" I asked, thinking of my grandfather's third wife and now widow. I don't remember what my parents said, but I was thinking about her just as much as I cried for my grandfather and dad.

Elisha had the luck of attending his funeral because she was in Texas on a school-related archaeology excavation at the time. She said it was a lovely service, and it was good to see the family. If for anything, I wish I hadn't gone to Ireland that summer because I wish I had the chance to say good-bye to my grandfather and see my cousin for one last time before he died of a drug overdose that following spring.

I remember chain-smoking that night while my parents were in bed. I started smoking when I was fifteen but really only when I bummed a cigarette from a friend at school or a party. It wouldn't be until 2009 that I smoked regularly.

For the next couple of weeks, I shed about ten pounds by going on light walks with Elisha and avoiding beer. I managed not to purge since I got home, but the desire was all too consuming.

A few days later, my parents, Grey, and I went to the movies; and for some reason, I decided it would be wise to check my voice mail (normally, I only listen to them to get rid of the annoying notification).

I got a call from St. Mary's, informing me that they had room for me. It was a Saturday, and I found out I got the message two weeks before I checked the voice mail, and the rest of the weekend was torture just waiting until Monday business hours to call admissions.

"I was abroad in Ireland," I said breathlessly.

"Well, how was it?"

"It was quite lovely and an enriching experience," I said quickly, waiting for the woman to tell me what I wanted to hear.

"Well, we saved a space for you and were just about to call you again!" the lady said excitedly.

I wanted it, God help me.

St. Mary's College of Maryland

I think out of the four schools I attended, St. Mary's College of Maryland was my favorite despite during time attended, I experienced the worst of my eating disorder and went so out of control with it that I was figured out.

My eating disorder escalated out of control at St. Mary's for a few reasons that were tiny in comparison to what I went through at CCU. I mean, the stress and insomnia there were powerful (shown by the fact I almost committed suicide) whereas at St. Mary's, the stress and insomnia were curtailed by frequent de-stressing visits home and a little "syrup" to help me sleep at night. All-nighters in the library exhausted me to sleep long hours, and a new group of friends and a party here and there were welcome changes too.

Perhaps I felt fat from gaining weight in Ireland and it needed to come off. Perhaps I missed my old friend, purging. I think I fell into the worst of it because I finally realized I had no direction in life. I just declared my major, but I knew I would never become an anthropologist. I think I just chose it because it's a favorite subject, and I was just too stupid to study any other subject.

Anyway.

For all the physical and historical riches of the campus, nothing appealed to me more than the anthropology department of St. Mary's. It was well put together, and the professors were kind and engaging. And it just so happened that the department had split with the sociology department, due to some contention, and they were reworking the course catalogue, which benefited me greatly.

My first class was anthropology research methods, and we spent the first two hours introducing ourselves and sharing with the class what relevant coursework or associations we had within the field of anthropology.

"Hi, I'm Jessica," I began awkwardly (sometimes I fucking stumble over my words, and I did so here). "I took an introductory course in anthropology at Montgomery County Community College, studied the historical and modern-day Irish culture this past summer, and I'm the student board member/liaison of the Washington Association of Professional Anthropologists."

WAPA is an organization of anthropologists along the East Coast, mainly in the DC region and tristate area. A meeting is held once a month where we all gathered in DC to discuss a topic of particular interest. My particular job was to be the bridge between professionals and students, make students aware of WAPA, and check the site's e-mail. It is thanks to my advisor at Montgomery College for that position (and the lack of other student entries).

Well, it just so happened that my new professor was president of WAPA several years back, and he told my new advisor who then asked for a meeting with me a couple days later.

"As you may have heard, the anthropology department split with the sociology department, and we are in need of an anthropology club. I'm certain the sociology club members won't be too happy about it"—if I recall correctly, it was still the socioanthropology club—"and you might have some problems with SGA approving of it, but I was wondering if you would be up for the task of organizing it."

I looked at my advisor with awe. "I would be delighted" I informed her in a sober tone that refused to give away my elation for having been chosen. It would turn out that my friends and I did get some lip from the sociology club members, one of whom was an SGA board member who wouldn't stop flapping her freaking gums about it. My new friend, Mary, had the gift of shutting her up quickly and winning over the board, and we were given our club.

I should say that others after me would have done a better job running the young club even though I gave it my all in between a shitload of course work and making ourselves known to the campus community. Corey, my senior year housemate and great friend, certainly proved better as the president than I, and I'm overjoyed that he managed to gain the club's popularity two years after we started it and all the while being the president of another club.

My first year at St. Mary's proved to be harder than I thought. I knew it would be hard and the classes demanding, but it seemed more than I could handle, and the pressure caused me to break.

February 19, 2009

I'm sick of being a size four. I'd like to get to my size 0's that are waiting patiently in the bottom drawer back in my room.

Right now I am sitting in the library, trying to complete this paper but I am instead gazing out at the choppy waves of the river. It is cold outside and I wonder what it would feel like to just wade out into the active frigid waters. Is that suicidal?

I want to drive to this one cool spot down the road where it's fun to spin out but I'm sure I'd do something stupid to myself out there. And my car. But more so me.

April 6, 2009

Starving myself and purging with more frequency.

I threw up tonight and just like every time, I remember how much I hate it. Took about three minutes to get it coming too because I had second thoughts.

More blood.

Rosie knocked on my door and asked if I was okay because she heard me hacking my brains out. My eyes were red and puffy and my nose runny. Lovely, right? I told her I just choked and had the sniffles.

"Oh. Well drink some water." She said before proceeding to tell me about her tarot card reading reveal.

April 10, 2009,

Purged again.

I came home today and Grey and I decided to get sushi with Elisha and Carissa. Dinner was very pleasant. I got the rainbow roll, allowed Grey to eat three of them while picking the fish and cucumber out of the rice and nori, and subsisted on that and a diet coke. But then I had one of Grey's spider rolls and immediately felt greedy and greasy. I needed to purge.

I went inside and discovered that the one bathroom door was locked.

Fuck! Don't people realize that I am on a mission to STARVE MYSELF? HOW AM I TO LOSE WEIGHT IF I CAN'T GAG THIS SHIT UP???

I waited two minutes but somebody was really having a ball in that bathroom. I walked outside again, dejected. Luckily we were all finished and decided to walk to Starbucks to chit chat.

Their slow steps really pissed me off and it felt like an hour rather than five minutes getting there. To my happiness, the bathroom was empty and I jammed two fingers down my throat and purged.

"What's wrong?" Asked Carissa.

"I sneezed."

Gosh, what's with the interrogation?

"It is the season." Elisha agreed.

Grey just looked at me. I'm not sure if he knew but he didn't say anything. He's probably just tired of dealing with it.

Earlier today, I walked in the front door, pet the cats, and said hello to my parents. I was wearing a nice slimming outfit. My parents told me that Elisha was in the basement and my dad followed where he began cutting paper on the long cutting board in the other room.

Elisha and I exchanged hugs where after she remarked "You lost weight!"

"Shh!" I hissed.

I've become very paranoid that my parents might discover my issues run deeper than body dysmorphic disorder.

April 11, 2009

Over breakfast this morning I found myself restless to return to school where I can consume 100 calories over the span of several hours. Not 15 minutes.

Today I am picking up Damon, my cousin, from GWU. I'm so excited! I love seeing Damon because he's like my best friend. It makes me happy that he's going to school in DC because I can see him more often.

Goddammit, I was painting my nails in the basement, walked upstairs to put away the varnish, and walked into the kitchen where Carissa was baking a coconut cake and my mother, lasagna. I was more than a bit puzzled because we were planning on going out to dinner.

"It's for Damon to take back to school." My mother explained.

"Yeah, your mom is happy to be cooking REAL food. For someone who will actually EAT it!" My dad chimed in.

I laughed uncomfortably. My mom always tries to send food back to school with me to at least give to my roommates. I don't like to take it because I get tempted to eat it. Or if I don't, I get jealous that someone else will enjoy it.

It's actually pretty amusing that my dad mentioned what he said because within our nuclear family, aside from Nathaniel who is now moved out, my mom is the only person to eat what I refer to as 'real' food on a regular basis.

April 18, 2009

I just discovered that my cousin Mason overdosed a few days ago. I'm pretty shaken up.

God I miss him!

What really sucks aside from losing a loving blood relative is the fact that a few of my friends died since last summer (one through suicide) and it makes me wonder if I'm next. 'Death comes in three's' is the saying.

I talked with Grey last night about my own issues and he agrees that my issues have gotten worse. After the exchange of words, I realized two things:

It must be one of the hardest and heaviest burdens to carry, watching your loved one hurt him/herself and Grey must be asking himself why do I deal with this?

I realized I need to be more careful with what I tell people. The thing is, you can pretend you have a little secret but it's not really a secret. People are very perceptive. My friend Clarice knew right off the bat that I had trouble eating, just like I knew she did. Fact aside that we both know the ropes of eating disorders and saw the signs with more clarity than others, it's pretty obvious if you look close enough.

This is why I'm hardly with my friends anymore. How do I tell them I'm not going to eat this or that because it will go straight to my thighs?

Mary and Kelly wouldn't understand. I hate that I have to keep myself from my closest friends but it's the only way to keep myself safe and thin.

May 28, 2009

Elisha leaves for Grenada in an hour. I'm jealous and will miss her.

My days seem pointless. The endless procession of minutes, hours, days . . . they seem to pass slowly and I am unconvinced that I as a person have anything to contribute to this world. My life is meaningless. All I can think about is my weight and food. And I look towards the future with tremendous fear because I see no direction.

I have dreams and desires for the future but it seems like a massive feat to acquire them. Fulfilling them will be one of the hardest challenges I have ever encountered and I am not so sure that I can go through such a task.

Louisa May Alcott once said or wrote, I don't really fucking know nor do I particularly care . . . "Far and away there in the sunshine are my highest aspirations . . . I may not reach them, but I can look up and see their beauty, believe in them, and try to follow where they lead . . ."

Once in my life I took solace in this but my belief in it now seems a bit dim. How can I see my own aspirations and believe in them if I don't believe in myself?

Recently I have found myself reflecting on my childhood with such yearning, and the present and future with such trepidation that I don't think I can cope with life. Being human is a great thing while one of the hardest burdens to bear. Sometimes I just want to check out. This is one of those moments. I'm not writing this to appear as though I am some fake angsty idiot college student complaining about the woes of the world. I am in serious pain and this is my only outlet.

I feel so forsaken and not even my prayers give me solace.

May 30, 2009
11:30 AM.

Binging. I feel so fat and gross. Want to puke but there are too many people in the house.

Thighs touch.

10:00 PM.

Continued binge. Purged. Ugh, ice cream does not come up right. Its cloying sweetness can be tasted from the pit of my stomach before it even reached my taste buds. But I won't complain. I was able to get it all up and I feel clean again.

12:30 AM, May 31.

Abusing sleep aids again but I guess it's better than drugs.

I hate myself so much. My thighs touch. All I want is to disappear.

I badly want to apologize to everyone I love. At some point in my childhood I had become the abnormality; my focus on food, diet, weight, looks . . . they are all I care about and I want my family to know I never intended for this to happen. I am not self absorbed or vain, or even trying to impress anyone. All I want is to shrink and disappear . . . to remove myself from the world and stay out of everyone's way.

I am such a burden.

I love you, Mom and Dad. I am so sorry.

I'm sorry, Elisha. I look up to you because you are so perfect, and you can never know of my failures.

I'm sorry Grey, because you dote on someone who is a total failure. Oh God, I'm so sorry.

8:30 PM

Had a pepsid. Heartburn was persistent all day. I hope it's not a side effect of my purging. My pulse feels funny too.

June 1, 2009

So I asked my mom if insurance paid for therapy or if she paid out of her pocket.

"Insurance." She replied soberly. "Why? Are you ready to go back?"
???

I thought she had forgotten.

My mother continued.

"Remember you always said you would continue looking after you saw that one woman—"

"Dr. Carlotta." I interrupted in a defeated grumble.

"Yeah . . . you shouldn't wait to get to a certain weight before you go back. It's not about that."

Yes it is! I wanted to scream. Instead, since the cat was apparently out of the bag, I said "I'm not ready."

"You can always choose to quit, Jessica." My mother said softly.

But I don't want to.

I think this journal entry chokes me up the most when I read it. My mother tried to tell me she knew something was wrong and that she wanted me to get help. How cruel fate has been to give her a mentally ill child and how cruel of me to ignore my mother's plea. I'm so sorry, Mommy.

June 7, 2009

I don't know how I have been so careless. My parents discovered that I've been binging and purging. Was I really that loud? Damn those thin walls and echo-y bathrooms!

Here's what happened. I wish I could be more eloquent but I'm too angry to articulate anything.

So I went up to my room and cried and my mother saw and heard my sobbing. "What's wrong?" She asked, shutting the door behind her.

I immediately wailed about my inefficiency as a person, that school was taking its toll on me, blah blah blah.

Mommy sat with me while I spewed all my fears and apprehensions and then she said "It's taking a toll on your body too, isn't it?"

SHIT.

I sobbed louder and harder. For some reason, I couldn't deny it. I nodded and continued to cry and say nonsensical shit.

"It gets worse when I'm stressed about school and gets better when I'm not."

"And it's easier to purge when you don't have roommates too?"

She had me all figured out. I sobbed more and gave myself a sobbing hang over.

If there could only be one thing to be embarrassed and ashamed about toward myself, it's the amount of crying I admit to. The eating disorder and self-mutilation are only guppies to what I feel about the crying.

June 7, 2009

My mother told me she and my dad heard me last night.

I couldn't lie to her. I'd be embarrassing the both of us if I lied.

I told her I had been purging and submitting to my demons since I was eight.

I swear, if I could have lied, I would have because the pained expression on her face made me cry harder and then she started to cry.

No. Stop it, Mom.

My family has a straightforward approach to pain and I rarely see my mom cry. It makes me uncomfortable to see her cry, probably more than worried or sad. I have no idea what to do, if anything at all.

I hastily and massively lied to her that I haven't purged much until this year, and I left out the bits about the drug abuse, the cutting, and a few other things.

As I said, we have a pretty abrupt and no nonsense 'what the hell do you expect me to do when it's your fault you aren't feeling well' rule to being sick in this household and it probably explains my unusually high tolerance to pain. If you are sick, ride it out. High fever? Pop a pill. Broke a bone or sprained a wrist or ankle? Get a cast. Need stitches? Get them. Need to go to the hospital? Just go and be done with it. However, it seemed an eating disorder was above all that and required TLC and a more thorough approach to getting well. I supposed you can't just say 'get over it' because it's more complicated than a cold.

I feel horrible and guilty for deceiving my family but I felt more fear than guilt about what was going to happen to me.

"Promise me that you will go back to therapy."

I wanted to die. I didn't want to go back to therapy that would help me open my eyes and leave me saying 'gee, golly! I don't need to be a size zero. I can eat normal and be a happy fat cow.'

My life is on lockdown now. How will I lose weight?

No. I have to keep my cool. They can't force me to stop exercising can they?

Later . . .

My mom apologized over and over again. She thinks she failed me. "I'm so sorry, Jessica. You were in so much turmoil for so long and I never saw it."

I hugged her. "How could you? I wear it on the inside and didn't want to burden you with it."

Took a laxative and swiped a perc.

May 8, 2009

My dad talked to me this morning before I left for work. So many thoughts coursed through my mind. I explained to him how it wasn't my ED speaking when I said I wanted to be thinner but he told me it was.

"I guess." I grumbled but still failing to see the connection.

My first appointment with my new therapist is July 1st. I'm not looking forward to it at all. Not. One. Bit. My mom gave me the option of having her present for the first meeting. Truth be told, I don't think I want her present in a meeting EVER. There is stuff I never even told Grey, and things I tried to deny myself.

New Friends and Support

Before I finalize this . . . memoir . . . . with journal entries of time spent in Residential Treatment, I want to explain that although I absolutely hated Residential Treatment, I LOVE the girls I spent my time with (most of them. Some just grated on me).

As a sarcastic bitch and a common loner, I tried distancing myself from the others at first, but being bonded with them by forces of self-destruction, eventually I cracked and accepted the fact that I needed them just as much as they needed me. Has this ever happened to me before? Being needed by someone? Perhaps Grey, but for once in my life, I sought the company and support of my kindred spirits and knew they would never push me away or make me feel negative about myself.

Even if one of us couldn't *stand* being in the presence of a particular patient, we never intentionally went out of our way to make them feel horrible because they already did that to themselves as we did to ourselves. Despite my feelings of Residential Treatment and recovery being bullshit, the "keep your chin up" attitude (from the patients, not the counselors) was a welcome change from hiding in the dark hole of our eating disorders and whatever other fucked-up issues had us so wrapped up in self-destruction. I've always been horrible in providing the "keep your chin up" advice, but sometimes, a hug and having them know you are there for them is enough.

We made promises of seeing each other when we left, and sometimes we did, if we lived close by or could afford the trip. I met up with two of the other girls once, but after that, with school, the crumbling tools for recovery, and the full blown return of my eating disorder, I shut them out except for the occasional phone call or "<3" message on their Facebook walls.

Now I truly wish I met up with them all as I promised because as I sit here in the dark, telling you about my damned issues, I only have the faintest memory of what their hugs felt like. Sitting in the same room with them. Gossiping about "the real world" outside of Residential Treatment. Bonding with them during episodes of *Glee* (I can't stand that show). Going shopping with our day passes. You know . . . things that friends do.

It's only now that I realize that despite having formed the tightest bond with these girls, I hardly know anything about them. Only today do I get glimpses of their lives, but unfortunately, through Facebook News Feed. I should chat with them more often. But I'm a socially awkward moron, and by that, developing a conversation would be more like handing out a questionnaire.

I may have mentioned making "best friends" in Residential Treatment (I could peruse what I had already written for you, but I'm too lazy to look back, other than for the purposes of editing), and I do still talk to them occasionally, and for hours sometimes; but there is a solid chunk of the other girls I talk to nearly every day now, and wish I developed a closer bond to them during our time together.

I have such an awesome support system here, with girls ranging in personality, ED's, and age. We have no cliques or prejudices and we are all genuine in our support for everyone to recover. There's Tilly, my Urban Outfitter and Free People Buddy from NY. She's gorgeous and hilarious and it's nice to talk to someone who is like me in personality.

Melody, who is so smart and quiet, but loud and firm in her commitment and with her support.

Kelly, the sweet Cali girl who I can unload my feelings to and likewise.

Jessa, sweet, smart, beautiful, and hilarious, whom I've known since my first day here and can relate to on nearly everything.

Kasey, the awesome, intelligent, gorgeous goof ball who is one of the most supportive ladies I have ever met.

Shana, my roommate, makes me laugh uncontrollably and gives the best pep talks. I hope I can move to the House with her if I am still in Residential Treatment.

September 15, 2009

On a lighter note, my roommate, Shana, and I are really connecting since we both got here. Nice funny chats. Our suitemate, Kimmy, had to go to the ER because her bloodwork was all whacky.

"I can't believe Kimmy isn't back yet." Said Shana.

"Where is she?" I asked.

"She's in the ER!"

"Why?" I asked in concern.

"The same thing Rhonda had to go for."

"Bloodwork?"

"Yeah, her phosphorous!"

"Oh no! Not the PHOSPHOROUS!" We dramatically wailed.

We went into a fit of giggles because we didn't know what that meant.

September 20, 2009

Past few days have been interesting.

Yesterday, Shana and I went out on pass to go to Target, Barnes and Noble, and to get dinner. We also went to DD's to grab some caffeine. And more at Barnes and Noble. We had diet coke (3 glasses each) at dinner. Our tolerance to caffeine had dropped and we were jittery on the precious syrup flowing through our systems.

We read contraband (diet books, ED memoirs) and joked around about the stupid entries in the Guinness Book of World Records. Really? Shockputs while wearing flippers?

At dinner we were pretty sure everyone thought we were psychotic lovers because we frantically discussed our food exchanges, frequently asked for the time (we weren't allowed cell phones and who the hell wears a watch?), and shared a pretty disgusting chocolate cake. Afterward, we drove back to our little prison and joked around some more to kill time before actually having to go back inside. I actually pissed myself because I laughed so hard. For one, she told me that Tums was like candy and I ended up spitting it out the window because it tasted like sour berries in chalk form. But we joked that we should lower the car top so people could see the two classy Tums chewing bitches.

Anyway, the nurses finally took my blood and I told them I wasn't going to drink any more Gatorade until I had the results of my blood work.

When we entered Residential Treatment, every girl was reminded that we would be living with and leaving with a support system of friends and family and our medical team. Voicing our thoughts to others is a tool for recovery, and regularly voicing these thoughts are supposed to lead us to our destination more expediently. My family is very supportive; never once had they shown me otherwise. And although I prefer talking to my Residential Treatment pals because they know exactly what's on my mind, it's important to talk to someone who isn't eating disordered, just for perspective.

I was astounded to see so much lack of understanding and support from some of the girls' families. It made me wonder how they treated their daughter's/sibling's success or lack thereof in areas that didn't pertain to an eating disorder. Having had full support from my own family, it was a new thing for me to have someone staring down at me as they walked past. Even though I already believed myself to be worthless, it angered me to the point of seeing red when I would hear the verbal abuse my new sisters received from their family.

I won't say I was her knight in shining armor, because that wasn't my intention when I finally blew up on a young teenage girl's father when the girl began hyperventilating after something so appalling he said to her. I don't remember what exactly I said to him, but it went along the lines of "Who are you to dare speak to her that way when even you say you don't understand why she is the way she is?" Actually . . . I didn't *say* it to him. It was more like a launch of a rocket to space, or a new world record for breaking the sound barrier. It was an explosion of hatred for the man, and he was taken aback before he told me to mind my own business. "Fuck you," I said before walking away, not realizing I could have gotten the young girl into serious trouble.

Perhaps I exploded in the way I did because I usually don't care what I say around strangers, or perhaps I exploded because for so long I wanted to yell back at my own father, respond with the pent-up anger I felt when he targeted me with a cold shoulder, or falsely made accusation that I was too needy (again . . . I went out of my way to avoid my parents when I grew up, so stop raising that annoying issue you claim is true). All I required in the way of neediness was clothing on my back, food (weird, huh?), and occasional hug to be reminded I was loved. All of which was provided, but still, negativity sticks with you more than positivity, doesn't it?

I'm not at all blaming my dad for how I ended up, but I'm weak enough that the negativity sinks in harder. Sorry, Dad. You know me. You are a wonderful father, and you know the idiom "the apple doesn't fall far from the tree"? It's bullshit. I wish I could be more like you: inured to the harshness of living in a hectic world while still providing generous and kind love. Love you, Pops. You are my idol.

Back to Therapy

I returned to therapy, but this time specifically for the eating disorder and body dysmorphic disorder and to balance out my roller-coaster moods. I didn't particularly want to go back, and I'm sure you know why. I don't think my therapist knew about my suicidal thoughts and attempt, perhaps not even my psychiatrist because I kept those tidbits to myself for fear of ending up in a place for crazy people.

June 15, 2009

I just KNEW it would be one of those days when I woke up this morning, where the sadness is all enveloping. I cried as I drove to work, dwelled on the past and future, and wondered what it would be like if I jerked the steering wheel to send my car swerving into the trees. Spinning out would be fun, but not the rest of it.

July 2, 2009

I saw Dana, my new therapist, yesterday. It was an intense session, so much so that I am still stressed out. But I like her. She's nice, soft tempered, too engaging. Actually, I might not like her because of her kind nature. That's how they get to you.

Anyway, I went in there expecting a session every now and then but she suggested once a week. ONCE A WEEK! AND I have to see a psychiatrist, a NUTRITIONIST, and an internist! The nutritionist I am supposed to see for 'perspective' on healthy eating habits, and the internist to assess the damage I did to my body. I guess I don't mind the psychiatrist because these suicidal thoughts are literally killing me. I guess it's time to take some meds again.

I will tell you what though. If I have to start a calorie based meal plan that makes me gain an OUNCE of weight, I'm not seeing her anymore.

I can't write anymore. My arms are weak and I'm trembling.

July 6, 2009

I have to make doctors appointments today. I'm so nervous. How can I call in my family practitioner's office without hanging my head in shame? Two of my friends' mothers are nurses there and I don't want them to think I'm deluded because I've been ORDERED to request a battery of tests for my heart, esophagus, and blood, along with a complete physical.

And I certainly don't want to see a nutritionist about information I already know. I'm sure I could tell her a thing or two. The only appointment I looking slightly forward to is the psychiatrist. I need pills to kick this depression.

July 11, 2009

I turned 21 today. I am very unhappy and angry. I threw up last night and I wish I could have today because I ate like a pregnant whale.

Starting Monday I am going back on my diet. No breaks until my goal weight. These curves have got to go because I have three weeks until I head to the beach with Grey.

July 24, 2009

I saw Emma, my nutritionist, today. I like her but I don't like her approach. She suggested changes that I'm not ready to accept.

My new 'lifestyle' as she calls it, is a low glycemic diet. Eliminating wheats can help decrease stress levels and help out my adrenal glands, she says. I guess I like her holistic approach to the body, but I don't like how she thinks this meal plan (over 1200 calories) is appropriate and that at least ¾ of each meal must be consumed to do the body good.

The hell you say, lady. I may be fluctuating in weight right now, but I'm trying to lose it and introducing 1300 plus calories is not going to help!

July 27, 2009

Called the doc today and I'm so frustrated. My thyroid results came in and the nurse scolded me. "Your T4 levels are TOO high!"

Jesus. I had my labs checked in May and my T4 levels were too LOW. So they upped me to 90 ug. And how is this MY fault? Is it necessary to use that tone with me?

I also feel like I am in a game of tug of war. My dietician says I should get off cytomel and get on something called armour thyroid but the nurse snippily said "honestly! I don't know where these dieticians get their information. It only works in place of T4."

Fine. I'll listen to my doctor but it is quite ridiculous to be chastising me for my fluctuating thyroid levels.

It's also official that I am a fat pig. My LDL is high. I'm too angry to talk about the rest of my results.

July 28, 2009

It's official. Elisha and I are going to Greece in December for Christmas! We will be staying on an island called Paros, in the Cyclades. We fly into Athens on Christmas and then to the island on the 26th.

Gotta lose weight for this!

Anyway, I'm going to the Outerbanks in a week. I'm so angry at myself because I weigh 112 pounds.

Yoga after work.

August 11, 2009

Yesterday I came home from the Outerbanks. I had a lot of fun but my issues were more pronounced.

Obviously I had fun because it was the beach. Grey also took me antiquing (one of our favorite past times), took me to a very nice restaurant, we went see glass hunting on the sand (found two lovely pieces of perfectly pebbled red glass), we made mimosas and watched the sunrise on the beach . . .

But at the same time I found myself retreating to the mirror to see if I had gained any weight. I purged three times. I think it's because I consumed the amount of calories I needed in order to maintain my weight. That many felt foreign to me, felt too much and too many, seemed as though it went straight to my thighs . . .

It could also be because I was in a two piece bathing suit regularly which certainly made it impossible to hide my body. I felt like I was being judged.

August 14, 2009

Anyway . . . my parents' new skittish dog is sitting right next to me as I flip through the tv stations. You know, a lot of these Discovery Health shows are capable of putting the fear of God into anybody. I just finished watching 'Science of the Obese' and it pretty much did instill the fear of God into me.

A man who is 100 lbs overweight did nothing but consume 25 extra calories a day. That's how he gained weight? Why does my nutritionist want me to eat more!?

August 16, 2009. 1:00 AM

Barfed again. Knees and calves weak. Not particularly tired so I took two Tylenol PMs. Dizzy.

3:30 AM

Purged again. Popped some vessels around my eyes.

August 19, 2009

111.5 lbs. My hope is to be 110 in three weeks.

Today's session with Dana made me very emotional because she suggested Residential Treatment should be a consideration, and she asked me what I thought about that.

'Are you fucking kidding me?' I wanted to shout. But in truth, I honestly didn't know how to respond to her question. On one hand, it would be easier to for my treatment being under 24 hour watch and talking to trained professionals when I feel the need to, but on the other hand I find those reasons scary and more: meal plans that must be met with compliance and may result in weight gain, seeing girls sicker than me, exposing my emotions to those girls . . .

But I was pleased Dana thought I was sick enough to warrant a stint in rehab.

She asked me if I put together the list of my symptoms. I read them aloud. She 'confirmed' I was bulimic (I use quotation marks around 'confirmed' because there would be future dispute as to whether I was just bulimic or Eating Disordered Not Otherwise Specified. Later, I would be confirmed as the latter).

Dana saved about thirty minutes of the meeting to perform a psychotherapy session to help me focus on calmness and breath during my most anxious of moments. It was almost as though I had been put under hypnosis because I couldn't really move and the bluish color of the carpet I had been staring at seemed to separate in hues of greens, yellows, and purples.

I was asked to think of a place and I chose to hide away in thoughts of roaming evergreen forests and expansive icy lakes.

"Take note of how this place affects your senses. What is the smell? How does it feel?" Dana asked in a tone that seemed miles away, only carried to me by the wind in my hideaway.

I left the office feeling calm and I seemed to notice new things about the surrounding land as I drove home.

August 26, 2009

Let me tell you about a typical day in my life.

Mornings follow as thus: on a good morning, I wake up and lay in bed and my first thought is "what's the point of it all? Why bother getting up?" Eventually my new mood stabilizing medication would kick in and these feelings and thoughts pass relatively quickly. On a bad day it can take hours for me to move. I crawl out of bed and because I move too quickly, my vision slacks, I sway, I bang my head or knee on my night stand or topple over. Fucking blood pressure.

Then comes breakfast. A wonderful, glorious 110 calorie parfait not only good for me as it possesses all the macronutrients my body requires, but it is a safe food. On a good day I don't feel the need to throw it up. A bad day? I get on the scale which measures to the tenth of a pound and will see my weight has inched up two points and I feel like I don't deserve the parfait.

By lunchtime my BP worsens and I both love it and hate it. I consume lots of salt or sugar free electrolyte infused drinks to stay the dizziness and fatigue.

Early evening? I hate myself because I haven't exercised, I'm bored, and the kitchen beckons. I try to stave off hunger til dinner which is at 7:30 but some days I will hoard certain foods and binge and then purge and refuse dinner.

I am really scared by dinnertime. The food is so tantalizing that I eat more than originally planned. Like ¾ of what's on my plate. After that, I feel anxious but sometimes I can't throw up because I feel as though I'm being watched.

Bed time is the worst part of my day. Everyone is in bed and I am still wide awake, all on my own. I binge and purge, sometimes several times a night. When I manage to curb my habits, I can't sleep because my electrolytes are so imbalanced

Then it starts over.

Residential Treatment

If you couldn't tell, and as you will see, I wasn't a big fan of Residential Treatment. Every day was a struggle in so many ways. For one, I had to address my "issues" as a "problem" that "needed to be fixed." Secondly, I was with a large group of girls who reminded me of myself so much that I burned with hatred and disgust. Originally, I had distanced myself from them because of my disgust, but so quickly did I falter and accept their unwavering love and support. Third, in Residential Treatment, you are not to be trusted and are treated like a criminal on lockdown and watch, thankfully without the dogs and shotguns.

That third point about Residential Treatment is what leaves me pounding the keys in frustration and loathing. *Of cooouuurrrssseee* all of us were con artists, figured out (or confessed on own free will), and thrust into a home where the counselors or doctors rapped us on our hands and wrists to let us know that we are very, *very* bad. And I say it in such the way I did because some of the counselors, some of the nurses—such power play is unprecedented.

You don't see this shit in school or with older siblings. Not in relationships. I'm not saying that they were cruel, but the level of *shame* some of them forced upon us—at least me—is still burdensome to my everyday being. I can't help but think one of them will pop out of the woodwork and tell me I'm not recovering hard enough. They had their words and tone down to an art, to a *science*.

I found myself hiding behind some of the nice counselor's backs to avoid the shaming speeches the others would spit upon you during meals. Again, they weren't mean, but I don't think they really realized that their manners and methods weren't effective for me and some of the other girls. I'm not saying they should have super sugarcoated anything, but c'mon. After shaming *myself* for so long, a few hearts and rainbows would have been very welcome.

I'm not quite sure why their tone and manners affected me so. Perhaps it was because I never *had* someone shame me about my eating habits, and having it all sink in so short an amount of time took its toll on me.

I wasn't too fond of my first psychiatrist in Residential Treatment either. She kind of reminded me of me with my first job: not really caring, coming up with ideas and answers to pretend I cared, and rolling out at five because work was a hassle, and I honestly *didn't care.* Or maybe she did care but just sucked at her job.

Like most first psychiatric appointments, I was handed packets of forms to fill out, to assess the level/severity of my issues, and rather than follow up with questions, I was hastily diagnosed and labeled with things that even I—in my fucked-up state—know aren't even applicable to me. Even my therapists and other psychiatrists would agree.

During the day, all the girls were assigned certain tracks, kind of like classes, but all designed to address our issues. Some were mandatory, but others could be chosen from a list of sorts, or if there was space for an extra patient and if a certain amount of tracks were met for the daily track quota (as I call it).

Each girl's schedule was designed based on her psychiatric records that she was admitted for. Of course all were there because of an apparent eating disorder, but there were also matters of drug and alcohol abuse, body dysmorphic disorder, anger, trauma, self-mutilation—you name it. Then there would be art and writing tracks, meditation (always puts me to sleep because it was so calming), music, and I think maybe movement too to allow us a less emotional outlet in which we could address our issues and share our feelings.

Drug and alcohol abuse and body dysmorphic disorder tracks were assigned to me. I never let my self-mutilation be known before now, so that track wasn't assigned to me (also, if I did let them know, they would put my "sharps," like leg razor, nail file, what have you, into a container, so how would I be able to groom myself?), nor did I really address my anger issues to my psychiatrists or therapists. Trauma? I never *really* faced unfortunate traumatic events (at least I tell myself so to block out the necklace incident), so that was out too.

I went to my first drug and alcohol abuse session to humor my psychiatrist, but I got up five minutes through and left. It wasn't for me, I decided, because my issues with alcohol and drugs weren't nearly as dangerous as were the other girls' abuse and addictions. I was also afraid my dumb ass would blurt out I did abuse drugs, which would open a new can of track worms for me. So. That left body dysmorphic disorder tracks and tracks designed for Eating Disorder Not Otherwise Specified patients.

Creative writing, art, meditation, music—I really only opened up in these tracks because I really only open up through creative forms of expression. Unless in one of my mandatory tracks one girl would open up about an event or issue that hit so close to home (and I would cry like a little bitch because of it and thus be annoyed by the track leader to share with the other girls why it affected me so), my feelings were mostly shared on paper and through sound. I still have some of the creative writing pieces tucked somewhere in a shoe box, and some of the art hangs on my bedroom wall. One picture hangs on some wall in the Residential Treatment house and was also copied into one of their calendars.

The first two days were awful. I didn't even get to say bye to my mom, it took forever for me to be able to call Grey, I certainly *felt* like I was in rehab and a hospital for the mentally unstable, and the change in environment was unsettling.

Naw, this will be like college, I tried to convince myself. *An all-girls college . . . full of eating disordered girls . . . no . . . this is going* to *fucking suck.*

Day four felt like two weeks. Twenty-eight days felt like six months. So many emotions were poured out from myself and the others, and I likened it to blood gushing out of a slit throat, and that forced the minutes to drag out like hours and hours like days. Afternoons spent sitting around also dragged out the days because leisure time meant playing cards, assembling puzzles, and (I shudder) . . . knitting. There were other activities I'm sure (sometimes the art room would be open), but I would sit with the other girls and enjoy our conversations.

I had the same amount of ups as downs in Residential Treatment. Making friends, being able to breathe and relax (surprisingly) from zero tests and homework and class readings, living in a populated area where there is a large mall and a plethora of restaurants to choose from while out on pass—these were actually big pluses for me.

Having tried to avoid making friends and pushing myself *away* from already-made friends—it was a welcome change to be accepted and already unconditionally loved by these wonderful girls. The break from tests and homework were wonderful because after bogging myself down with classes that thrust me further into my issues, it was quite nice not having to spend all-nighters in the library. The mall is a definite given because I'm a girl who likes to shop.

That's all I can really say about Residential Treatment. I tried blocking it from my memories, except for the "tools for recovery" (which was mostly support system, in my opinion) and new friends.

August 28, 2009

> *I'm getting help. I'm not going back to St. Mary's this semester. I don't know yet whether I will be put in residential or outpatient treatment. I'm going to miss my friends so much. I'm depressed that I have to miss my Food and Culture course this semester.*
>
> *I remember telling Dana on Wednesday that I felt my dad perceived me as too much: excessive, needy, talkative. Today was a perfect example.*
>
> *Well, my mom and I were getting the ball rolling with residential when my dad had walked in the front door. Well great, now my dad needs to know because I told my mom two minutes ago I'd be in the office.*
>
> *I walked into the office where my parents were and unloaded the unfinished business to my mom because I was supposed to tell her when I finished talking on the phone with Philly's top dogs. My dad looked at me and I told him I wasn't going back to school.*

'I know. We will talk about this later.' He said in a very tight and clipped tone.

Later he told me he was just busy. Why did he allow me in the office if he was busy? And he told me he thought 'it had to be all about me.'

I found this to be incredibly hurtful. I told him that's not why I came into the office. I ALWAYS WENT OUT OF MY WAY TO AVOID THEM. I NEVER WANTED TO BE AROUND.

HOW ABOUT I JUST NOT FUCKING GO TO REHAB, DAD? I DIDN'T WANT TO IN THE FIRST FUCKING PLACE NOR DO I NOW AND IF IT WILL HAVE YOU STOP SAYING THAT BULLSHIT I WON'T GO. IN FACT, I WAS PLANNING ON LEAVING THE FUCKING EAST COAST ANYWAY SO I'LL JUST GO AHEAD WITH THOSE PLANS.

I think I'm calm now.

I don't like how he jumps to conclusions. Sometimes I wish I still had a nanny because they listened to me and passed no judgment, no matter how much of a terror I could be to them. I know they loved me.

I'm going to St. Mary's tomorrow to visit my friends and talk with my advisor.

September 1, 2009

I'm really fucking mad. About everything. I'm sitting in Medical Access because I couldn't make a doctor's appointment with my family practicioner and I needed an appointment ASAP because Residential Treatment cut my time short in terms of my assessment appointment. It would have been easier if my mom were with me.

I'm pissed because upon seeing my supportive friends and advisor, I feel like I made the wrong decision in taking medical leave.

I'm pissed because I'm being treated like a lab rat and a mental patient. All eyes are on me because 'she's eating disordered!'

September 2, 2009
MIDNIGHT

I'm so dizzy. This is the worst I've felt after purging. My vessels popped again and my knees feel like they've been weighted with lead. I could pass out right now. But it seems impossible.

4:00 AM

Purged again . . . strange there are no weak feelings.

I had my medical assessment today and my 'team' is reaching a decision as to whether I will be attending partial treatment in Bethesda or residential in Philadelphia.

I hate Bethesda. Such a depressing city. It's too far a drive and too institutional.

September 6, 2009

I'm going to Philly on Wednesday. Don't know for sure my arrangements so I'm not even sure why I need to drive 3 hours up to that damned city rather than hear it over the phone.

Speaking of the 'phone', I had a phone consultation with Jill, a representative, and she was asking me for a list of symptoms, behaviors, and weight history. I told her everything and she flummoxed me by asking if I had been in treatment when I had weighed 98 pounds.

'That weight is too low for a person of my height?' I blurted. I wasn't exactly knocking on death's door. Come to think of it, I didn't even KNOW I had an eating disorder when I was at 98 pounds. Regardless of the purging, I wasn't anorexic (I don't think? Maybe I would have been subtyped) which in my mind seemed to be the only eating disorder out there. Silly me for not knowing that a consistently low calorie diet, constantly counting the calories to the EXACT NUMBER, and feeling guilty about exceeding 1200 are all behaviors of an eating disorder.

September 10, 2009

It is day 2 in Residential Treatment and I already want to go home.

I haven't had but three hours of sleep in the past two days and I feel heavy. I stepped on the scale for the second time at 4 AM and I am convinced that these sadists want every girl to gain weight, regardless of her set weight. I think they should personalize meal plans because I know for a fact that weight gain is a cause for relapse and resistance to treatment. If I gain weight, I am getting it off right when I leave this place, healthy or not! Most of the girls told me they had gained weight and I can't tell if they are anorexic, bulimic, subtyped, binge eating, or eating disorder not otherwise specified.

I was orthostatic this morning, and yesterday. The nurses force me to drink Gatorade within five minutes and tell me I have to do this for four more days until they know if I am naturally orthostatic or just need to replenish lost electrolytes. And I have to drink this shit during snack time too. To make matters worse, I have to pee a lot but because I'm under watch, my bathroom is locked and I have to ask a nurse or counselor to unlock it when I need to go. It's humiliating how some of them watch (to make sure I'm not bowing my head between my legs to purge . . . never done that. I still have my limits), or even when they have the decency to turn away but still engage me in conversation to make sure I'm not purging.

Belinda, the medical practicioner who is hardly ever around, told me I had a sinus arrhythmia but this is a normal abnormality that I should keep tabs on. 'Abnormality' and 'keep tabs on' don't sound so 'normal' to me. But I guess I shouldn't bitch and moan because she's the doc and some of these other girls have serious heart conditions.

I meet with my therapist today. I want to ask for computer and phone time because I need to talk to Grey because I miss him so much that it hurts.

Oh, met with my psychiatrist today and she thinks I have a problem with alcohol. As if I abuse alcohol to numb the pain as she suggests. I drink it to be social!

September 11, 2009

God Bless America.

I was told to write happy poems because my therapist and psychiatrist think I write too many daunting and hurtful things about myself. I need to mediate and seek out others. Try not to stress about meals or write about the stress.

Jesus . . . this is bullshit.

I really hate this food they force me to eat. I'm probably acting like a total snob but it's all grease! How does this support the USDA guidelines??? If I don't eat this slop, I'm told I have to drink an entire supplement, even if I leave behind a tiny cherry tomato.

I am already so full. Had to drink another bottle of Gatorade to rid the Ortho. But I'm so full that I just gagged on acid and bits of undigested food.

How . . . how is this healthy? These really are large portions and I'm not saying that as someone who hardly eats a big meal. There is dairy (milk or yogurt, usually) to be consumed. Protein. Fats. Carbohydrates. Fruit. Vegetables. I'd be so lucky to get a slice of pizza to account for the fat, protein, and carbs, just to make room for the other stuff. Or give me a smoothie! Smoothies have pretty much EVERYTHING in them, from the macronutrients to the micronutrients.

If I am this uncomfortable, how would forcing myself to eat all this healthy shit in one sitting three times a day help me if I had to force myself to eat even tiny amounts of food during my fasts, and forced myself to purge *during my binges? What they put in front of me three times a day is what I consider to be a binge.*

On a lighter note, I suppose I am making fast friends.

September 12, 2009

Anyway, about twenty minutes passed when I got back to my room and I 'slipped' and exercised for about five, walked the building for three, then sought help. I caved and sought a counselor. She was very sweet and attentive as I told her I feel like my inner core is thawing but I don't want it to.

I don't want to see my parents tomorrow. This place is an embarrassment and I just want to be left alone.

September 14, 2009

I hate this place. I gained a pound. 'Weight maintenance' and 'water retention' my ass. I can see the weight in my upper arms, my waist, and my hips.

Two sessions of art therapy today. Went to the first. 'If you could picture your hunger, what would it look like?'

I drew myself as Persephone who ate the pomegranate seeds and is trapped in the Underworld, forced into submission by Hades.

4:30 PM

Wow, only five days and already some progress! Moved up to Interdependent Eating! I'm excited about being moved to a different room but also nervous. I'm used to them portioning everything out for me and I'm scared about picking out the portions for myself because I suck at math and what if I get in trouble?

Also had therapy today. Maria thinks I should stop looking at the scale here, and when I go home I should only weigh myself during therapy or nutrition appointments.

Blah blah. I agreed just to get out of there because she granted me computer time but they coincide with my sessions! The only availability is Friday and that's four days from now. Three more weeks of this place sounds dreadful because this first week already feels like it's been forever.

I can't wait to see the leaves outside turn to gold.

I'm too scared to step on the scale in the morning.

September 15, 2009

I'm in such an up and down fluctuation of moods that it's driving me mad. Meal time makes me anxious, as do vitals and there are so many sessions and appointments that I feel like I am not allowed to slow down. The counselors and 'team' tell me to take it easy but I get penalized when I take it easy. So . . . how exactly am I supposed to take it easy?

I really want to go home and I even voiced it in community meal support or whatever it's called. I still don't know. But everyone gave me so much support and praise that my spirits lifted even though I HATE praise. They told me how smart I am, how sad they would be if I left, and also that I "have only one body . . . if [I] left, my sick body would prevent me from doing the things [I] wanted to do."

Very insightful.

Just go out of my appointment with Maria. It was another intense session. I told her how much I disliked Residential Treatment, the weight gain, blah blah. She told me Residential Treatment is still the place for me to be, that outpatient isn't good enough. She seemed genuinely adamant that this was the only way that I would personally be able to recover (blech. THAT WORD). But I was so relieved when she told me that Blue Cross might cut me off soon. I was so relieved.

After my appointment, I called Mommy and told her how much I hated it here. She was very compassionate but told me she would be very disappointed in me if I came home before Blue Cross cut me off, and if it didn't at all.

I'm fucking Ortho again. But I'll be damned if I go to snack to down another Gatorade.

Dinner was a freaking mess. It was a high calorie mess. I can feel the weight gain, especially in my waist and thighs where my jeans are getting a bit tight. When the nurses say my 'weight will eventually settle' I take that as a negative comment. I DON'T WANT IT TO INCH UP AND SETTLE GODDAMMIT. How could anyone love a person like me who carries so much negativity through the fat of her tummy and thighs?

I'm going to try to do the 'blind weighing'* tomorrow so I don't freak out on the scale.

---

*   Blind weighing: The nurses allow you the option of checking your weight on the scale or turning away from the flashing numbers. Blind weighing is the latter option, which is supposed to "empower" the patients.

September 16, 2009

Looked at the scale. Couldn't do the blind weights. Still 113.5. I hate this place. How can they be so cavalier about this fat settling around my midsection?

From 1:30-2:55 I was in a psychodrama session that made me so emotional. I hate showing others my vulnerable side.

Here's what went down: I picked a card from a deck that had a word and a picture that related to the word. Mine was 'fighting.'

I'm fighting so many things. My ED, gaining weight, my recovery, my body image . . .

I had to express this by selecting other girls to be characters and things relevant and central to my struggle with ED. Family, Grey, armor, ED, me, and my recovery. They all had to say what they meant to me and it had to pan out in what it would look like by the way I willed it. The voice of my ED was overshadowed by the voices of my other characters.

All I thought during that session was 'do I feel my jeans getting tighter right now?'

I called Pops and told him about my concerns, about how scared I was, and that maybe I was wrong, maybe I'm not ready to let go. I just want to be healthy but I don't want to have to gain weight and stop self mutilating in order to be healthy.

Anyway, good news! I'm off locked bathroom and watch and I moved upstairs with Shana.

I hope my vitals are okay tomorrow. I hope I'm not still Ortho.

Went to art therapy today and Sandy told me my drawing was amazing. Awesome, despite me hating praise. Anyway, the assignment went as follows:

"Have you ever heard anyone tell you that 'fat is not a feeling?' To which we all replied 'yes.' So we had to describe what we meant when she says we feel fat. I said "to me, feeling fat is a combination and excess of negative emotions that I feel are physically manifested through my appearance." I had NO idea if that made any sense to them. But we had to draw how we felt 'when we feel fat.'

I drew a candle sitting on a windowsill, separated from a raging fire by a single pane of glass. I am the fire, roaring with raging feelings, wanting to be on the inside with that calm candle flame.

Parents coming for a family session tomorrow.

September 18, 2009

I'm fuming. Still Ortho, still have to drink Gatorade, and the nurses lied to me. They said they'd draw my blood on the 6th day and it's the 8th. Whatever.

My day started out okay (except vitals) because I moved up to level four and am able to go out on pass tomorrow.

It really figures I would be sick the night before I go out on pass. I've been feeling ill all day. Dizzy, incoherent, stiff and shaky, and it worsened in Multiple Family Group.† The room was so stifling and hot. I thought I was going to pass the fuck OUT. Vicky (counselor) walked me to the nurse's station and even before I entered the station, they thrust a Gatorade into my hands and gave me two excedrins.

Um . . . THANKS FOR THE FUCKING HELP. Because you know, there's like . . . no need to check if it's something serious.

September 24, 2009

The House‡ is the Wynn compared to the motel-ish residence building.

HOWEVER, it was a bloody awful day. I was dropped a level because of a little misunderstanding that will not be stated. SO, I was not allowed to go on pass because of what they found during room searches.

Okay. THEY ARE IDIOTS since they haven't found it on day one. I mean, yeah, I deserve not to go out on pass. It's my own fault. But fuck this. THEIR RULES ARE SUFFOCATING. AND NO ONE TOLD ME I WAS DROPPED A LEVEL until 20 minutes before family therapy. So my parents drove this fucking far for a tiny 60 minute session?

I don't think my parents have ever seen me shout with such gale force. I am never rude to anyone unless they piss me off (which now that I think about it . . . it's pretty often). Maria is a calming therapist but I was so enraged.

---

†   Multiple Family Group: sessions held with family members present to express their own concerns, confusion, or support.

‡   "The House" I mentioned, is exactly what it sounds like. It is a house on the Residential Treatment grounds where girls 18 and over move into in order to transition them back into the real world. There was less monitoring (but equal amounts security) and once a week (or was it two weeks?) we would prepare from scratch our lunch. Some track sessions would exclusively be held for us at the House and the small group was more welcoming to me than seeing a larger group of my counterparts.

Living in the House also meant what I refer to as therapy field trips. They weren't really therapeutic, but they were meant to lend us perspective. There was one such field trip where we headed out to the grocery store to compare our "safe foods" with our fear foods. Shauna and I picked out what we feared most, and it did nothing to calm us.

Anyway, to provide light humor and perspective, here is an online conversation I had with Shauna when we were planning my trip to visit her up in Connecticut:

Shauna:

I know this is weird to bring up, but do you think we should just like hit up the grocery store together or I could pick up a few things before you get here? I think playing it by ear is a good way to go

Me:
Lets go to the grocery store. We should do that.

Shauna:

Thats a good idea I think too. greed.

Me:

We will be the windowlicking psychos shopping around, biting our fingernails while everyone stares haha.

Shauna:

Haha. I knowright emember our shopping trip we all had to take at Residential Treatment together

Me:

ahahahaha yes
My knit brows trying to pick out some cereal?
I felt like such a moron.
I need to include this conversation in on a section of my book haha. If you don't mind.

Shauna:

Not at all, I'd be honored actually.

I know, I remember the hardest part at the store was when they made us choose something we never allow ourselves to eat, and I freaking chose potato chipslollike the hardest thing to put down

Me:

he ice cream was the hardest for me. And I took it back to the House. And I loathed eating it.

Friend: Shauna

Ah, ice cream :/eah, I remember bringing mine back to the House too . . .

Needless to say, ice cream and potato chips are fear foods.

September 26, 2009

> *Today was hot and cold. It started out great: I went to art, went on an outing with the House group, and went on pass with Shana. But it was somewhat strained with Shana and it pretty much was my fault.*
>
> *First of all, I get really nervous when eating in front of strangers and that would have been Shana's family. I didn't eat at their house, which riled Shana. On the drive back I had a Clif bar and she told me about how I could make up the exchanges at snack time. I informed her that I appreciated her concern, but I am responsible for my own recovery, and tonight was just one little slip.*
>
> *I honestly am bearing through this 'exchange system' but it really sucks. I know I won't adhere to it for long once I leave this place. I don't know why I feel I have to keep justifying my actions when they are my own and I am my own responsibility.*
>
> *I mean . . . I'm not barfing anymore, am I?*
>
> *Anyway, Shana's family was very nice.*
>
> *Grey visits tomorrow. I'm embarrassed by what he will see and it will finally sink in for him that I really am psycho.*

September 27, 2009

> *My parents surprised me with a visit so they joined Grey and me to Chestnut Hill and dinner. We walked around the shops on Germantown Ave*

and drank coffee in Starbucks. We talked about what comes after Residential Treatment . . . maybe day treatment in Bethesda. I just want a job.

September 28, 2009

Feeling pretty low today. Body Image is pretty shitty and my mood worse. I want to isolate[§] myself today. I hope this is just my stupid period coming on. I pity the girls who come across the dragon that is me and my bleeding vagina.

September 30, 2009

Weight: 114
Shana and I went out on Pass yesterday. It's just really nice to escape from time to time.

October 3, 2009

WELL THAT WAS A TERRIBLE FAMILY SESSION.
This is what happened: Maria told me to express my greatest fear, the one thing I am scared my parents could do. So I told them that I am scared they don't see the severity of my eating disorder (despite now paying out of pocket for me to stay) and that one day they would stop caring as much as they do now.
Now . . . I am in no way an expert in articulating myself on command, and at that moment I said I thought maybe they'd lose faith.
Well. My dad went APE. SHIT. I actually hyperventilated through the whole thing. I couldn't wait to rush out of there and for the first time, I was happy to be in Residential Treatment where visiting hours were limited and I could storm the fuck away.
Tonight was a bunch of fun. A few of us . . . . drum roll please . . . WENT TO THE MALL. Oh how I missed clothes. The shopping for clothing. OMG. Free People. Shoes. Jewelry. OMG . . . just the walking is amazing. I'm pretty certain everyone thought we were fugitives because we acted so strangely.
Jenna and I went to get candy, which is a contraband item. Got me some muthafuckin' black cherry warheads. WHADDUP. It's sad how they were so much better than the dessert items we are forced to eat during mealtimes.

---

§   Isolate is a term used to describe a patient avoiding the company of others instead of reaching out to ask for advice or to talk their way through the issue.

October 6, 2009

Today is my last full day here.

October 7, 2009

I made a mistake. I need to be here. Why didn't I take Residential Treatment seriously?

I really should have taken Residential Treatment seriously because every purge, every fast, they all take their toll on me. I could end up with a heart disease later in life, or a fucking feeding tube. But it is really hard to quit especially when you tell yourself, "I'll start working on it tomorrow" and keep pushing it back. That's how I do it. I save things for the last minute, but the last minute may be too late this time.

My first relapse occurred just after Christmas 2009 and lasted a solid year. There were brief periods of peace here and there in between lapses and short relapses after that.

Having an eating disorder is not at all fun. I used to think it was a great thing because it ensured I would lose weight and I had something to control about myself. I thought it would solve all of my problems.

I repeat: an eating disorder is not fun. An eating disorder does *not* solve all your problems. It *gives* you *more* problems.

An eating disorder is a demon. Because it haunts you. And you believe in it and you think it is normal. But it isn't. And people will tell you that these things you are seeing and feeling aren't normal. These things you believe in are torturing you, sending you to madness, and they slowly kill you. And when the heart of your sanity stops beating, this demon drags you straight to hell, and nothing can save you. You should have exorcised that demon. Or at least repented because once you go in as deep as I have, there is nothing in this world that will keep you from falling deeper.

Perhaps if I actually listened in Residential Treatment, my view would be different. But I have been worn, embittered, and welcomed into the morbid nature of the world and on cold days . . .

It's pretty cozy living in my disturbing little universe.

Epilogue

Like so many times, before my lack of judgment has gotten me in trouble, I had hoped that perhaps I might reach that one glowing realization that all of this is nonsense and I very well *could* love myself.

I was so fucking wrong. SO FUCKING WRONG. So wrong in fact, that I have lapsed and relapsed on numerous occasions during this hellish process. I had to take several breaks from writing my story because reviving my history was too titanic and dangerous for me to do so soon after Residential Treatment. This proved to be too detrimental to my recovery.

Only a few years after Residential Treatment, I am still on the road to recovery. I don't think I will ever be labeled "recovered" or believe in a full state of recovery.

These days, I have stopped abusing painkillers and unprescribed sleep aids and severely curbed the amount of alcohol that I ingest. I weigh 105 pounds, eat as much crap as I do healthy foods, do yoga, and go for the occasional hike through the woods. I'm too scared to get back into heavy exercising and too scared to stop counting calories; but at least my fasting, binging, and purging habits are quickly diminishing. And I am somewhat cognizant of what happiness and health can be. Or maybe this is just one of those rare episodes where I begin to feel good about myself before the next lapse. Not sure. I try not to worry.

I shredded the pages of my journals and burned what remained, hoping that somehow, my past will go up in smoke with the pages. Yet I still find myself unconsciously reaching for pen and paper to write down a secret message to myself, an unhappy thought, or hurtful words that are supposed to make me feel guilty enough to shed weight. Then I shred those too and lose sleep over it.

The scale sits in the corner of the room for weeks at a time, collecting dust until I catch a glimpse of my body in the mirror and finally give in enough to wait for the blinking numbers to tell me what I so hate. Then I will lovingly replace the scale and crawl into bed after turning off the lights and hiding myself beneath the covers.

Sometimes, I find myself absentmindedly rubbing my wrist or tracing the faded calluses and scars on my knuckles and backs of my hands, wishing the marks would return to full pigmentation. Loyal indicators of my control slowly disappearing.

During the course of writing this waste of paper and computer screen space, spending time in the past through my memories and endless journal entries, the nightmares resurfaced; and I find myself again in the grips of insomnia. I lie awake in bed, during the witching hour, waiting for the fires of hell to finally whisk me away. Then the sun's rosy fingers reach through the windows, and magically I fall asleep. I will be so lucky if I don't wake in a cold sweat, screaming aloud or silently a few short hours later because of a recurring nightmare.

It's all a nightmare, asleep and awake. I have only myself to blame and too much pride to continue asking for help.

And now, I share with you the last journal entry I hope to ever write.

August 18, 2012

>Slowly I am accepting my body's curves and imperfections. I am responding to my stomach's damnable requests to be filled with sustenance, though I find it tiresome and time consuming. My old jeans are mocking me. I'm sure of it.

>I find myself gasping for breath in this game of tug of war. Which side am I on? Health and pressure compel me to tug myself under the shade of what one would call self-confidence but the darker, more seductive side prompts me to grasp for dear hold on the side that will pull me darker into my abyss of self destruction. My palms burn and my grip aches. My feet are slipping. My knees are buckling. Soon enough I will have to let go and let my calluses heal.

>The moment I let go, I will miss the pain. Sweet and morbid torture is all I have ever known.

I didn't write all of this for you to feel sorry for me. Everything I said, everything I shared is everything I wanted to get off my shoulders. I felt like someone was standing on my chest for so long, and in writing this . . . some of that pressure has been lifted despite the hellish process. I just gotta stop crying about it and grow up. Solve these problems on my own and for real this time. Say "Fuck you!" to my woes and move on. Graduate to a state of which some would consider "normal."

Below, a genuine smile and rare confidence. I'm sure I could gain a little weight as 105 is a trigger for me, but whoa, whoa, whoa. One step at a time.

But the really neat thing is I don't think I look fat (astounding because I never liked full-body photos of me sitting because of the way my stomach folds), and for once, I don't think prettiness is connected with thinness.

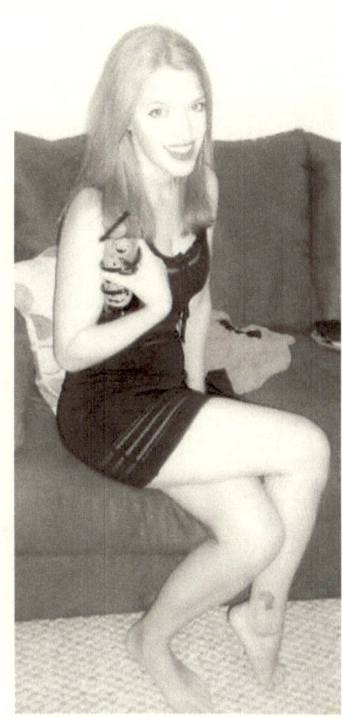

Date: October 31, 2012
Age: 24
BMI: 19.2
BMI range: normal

References

2000 Eating Disorder Diagnostic Criteria from DSM IV-TR 307.50 Eating Disorder Not Otherwise Specified. http://casat.unr.edu/docs/eatingdisorders_criteria.pdf, accessed October 28, 2012.

http://www.manicdepressive.org/dsm.html

(3.) http://www.ncbi.nlm.nih.gov/pmc/articles/PMC1978319/

www.ingramcontent.com/pod-product-compliance
Lightning Source LLC
Chambersburg PA
CBHW030355290526
45785CB00004B/1758